Statistics for Dental Clinicians

Statistics for Dental Clinicians

Michael Glick, DMD, FDS RCSEd
Professor and Executive Director
Department of Preventive and Restorative Sciences, and Department of Oral Medicine
Center for Integrative Global Oral Health
Cochrane Oral Health Collaborating Center
School of Dental Medicine
University of Pennsylvania
Philadelphia, PA, USA

Alonso Carrasco-Labra, DDS, MSc, PhD
Associate Professor, Department of Preventive and Restorative Sciences
Center for Integrative Global Oral Health
Cochrane Oral Health Collaborating Center
School of Dental Medicine
University of Pennsylvania
Philadelphia, PA, USA

Olivia Urquhart, MPH
Instructor, Department of Preventive and Restorative Sciences
Center for Integrative Global Oral Health
Cochrane Oral Health Collaborating Center
School of Dental Medicine
University of Pennsylvania
Philadelphia, PA, USA

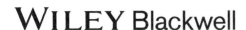
WILEY Blackwell

Published by John Wiley & Sons, Inc., Hoboken, New Jersey.
Published simultaneously in Canada.

For general information on our other products and services or for technical support, please contact our Customer Care Department within the United States at (800) 762-2974, outside the United States at (317) 572-3993 or fax (317) 572-4002.

Wiley also publishes its books in a variety of electronic formats. Some content that appears in print may not be available in electronic formats. For more information about Wiley products, visit our web site at www.wiley.com.

Library of Congress Cataloging-in-Publication Data applied for
[PB ISBN: 9781119810162]

Cover Design: Wiley
Cover Image: © Michael Glick, Alonso Carrasco-Labra, and Olivia Urquhart

Set in 9.5/12.5pt STIXTwoText by Straive, Pondicherry, India

SKY10052478_080323

To our past, present, and future students and mentors.

Contents

Preamble

During the past decades, we have had the opportunity to conduct research and publish in the biomedical literature. We have also had the opportunity to teach statistics and epidemiology to a range of academicians, clinicians, residents and students. Based on these experiences we have realized the need to better understand and interpret the scientific literature. This is more important today than ever before because of the ease of accessing the enormous number of scientific materials being published every day.

This book is not intended to teach readers how to conduct research or perform statistical analyses. Instead, this book is written for those who are interested in understanding and interpreting the biomedical literature to inform clinical practice. Twenty chapters cover basic concepts ranging from a general understanding of statistics to more complex topics, such as meta-analysis and regression analysis.

We realize that one of the most challenging areas in statistics is its very specialized language and jargon. In this book every statistical concept is explained in plain English, both within the chapters and in a separate glossary. For ease, most of the italicized words in the chapters can also be found in the Glossary. We have also attempted to minimize formulas and equations within the chapters, but for those who want a more in-depth understanding we have added an appendix where we provide equations and formulas for all the "numbers" we discuss in the chapters.

Other opportunities for the more curious reader are sections in most chapter entitled "a few additional notes," which complement the text, as well as suggest additional topics for those who are interested in gaining a further understanding. Furthermore, selected readings accompany each chapter.

Every chapter also has "Pullout boxes." These sections offer non-scientific examples or analogies that we believe provide simple illustrations of concepts discussed in the chapters. We have also included numerous tables and illustrations to serve as aids to facilitate the interpretation and application of the discussed statistical concepts.

We hope this book will help clinicians to inform clinical practice for the benefit of our patients.

1

What is statistics and why do we need it?

Paraphrasing from H. G. Wells's *Mankind in the Making* (1903), where Wells wrote, "The time may not be very remote when it will be understood that for complete initiation as an efficient citizen of one of the new great complex worldwide States that are now developing, it is as necessary to be able to compute, to think in averages and maxima and minima, as it is now to be able to read and write," S. S. Wilks, in his presidential address to the American Statistical Association, declared, "Statistical thinking will one day be as necessary for efficient citizenship as the ability to read and write." Moving forward 70 years, this statement has never been more relevant or germane.

Claims are made constantly about miracle cures for cancer, diets that promise 20-pound weight loss in one week, daily wine consumption either adding years to one's life or ushering in an early death, medication A lowering blood pressure better than medication B, toothpaste X cleaning better than toothpaste Y, and so forth. What to believe? Being able to understand and interpret the basis for these and similar claims is an important skill that many of us lack but can easily learn.

We are inundated with a vast array of scientific publications, easily available to anyone with a computer and internet connection. However, more is not always better, as many articles present diverse and, at times, contradictory information that must be appraised and interpreted to inform clinical practice. Data by themselves are not very useful and must be analyzed to generate meaningful information, which then needs to be further contextualized to a particular clinical setting and a patient's condition and need. An understanding of how data from scientific articles are generated, analyzed, presented, and interpreted has become essential to the informed clinician. This is where statistics comes in.

Statistics is essentially the scientific language the purpose of which is to describe, understand, and communicate scientific findings. An understanding of this language is needed to critically read, interpret, and understand the biomedical literature, with the ultimate goal of using scientific information for making informed decisions about etiology, diagnosis, prevention, treatment planning, prognosis, public policy, and much more. If statistics is a language, statistical concepts are the grammar (the rules of a language), while generation, organization, analysis, presentation of data, and the words used in this scientific language make up the syntax (the structure of sentences). Many statistical concepts can be similarly exemplified by using language as a comparison. For example, two important notions in statistics are *confounders* and *bias*. A confounder can be compared to a prejudice (known and unknown), while bias is similar to putting forth an argument but unintentionally using an incorrect definition (e.g., using usurping power when describing a democratic election).

Statistics for Dental Clinicians, First Edition. Michael Glick, Alonso Carrasco-Labra, and Olivia Urquhart.
© 2024 John Wiley & Sons, Inc. Published 2024 by John Wiley & Sons, Inc.

This book does not cover how to apply and perform statistical analyses but instead focuses on the understanding and interpretation of statistical concepts used in clinical research that are meaningful to health care professionals. An understanding of statistics, like learning a new language, starts with a grasp of commonly encountered statistical terms and concepts.

One main obstacle to understanding statistics is the field's specialized terminology. Words used in statistics do not always have the same meaning as in everyday language and must be interpreted correctly. For example, in statistics a *population* represents all members in a group of interest, while a *sample* is a representative subset of a population. The word *risk*, often used in everyday language to refer to something that reflects a potential threat, in statistics has neither a positive nor a negative connotation and represents simply the *probability* for an *event*, whether desirable or undesirable, to happen. Another example is the word "error," which in statistical vernacular sometimes means "variation" but can also be used to illustrate a mistake. Statistical terminology is explained and defined throughout this book; most italicized words can be found in the glossary.

Statistics is a homonym, a word that is spelled and pronounced one way but has multiple meanings. Statistics is a **discipline** involved with the collection, organization, analysis, interpretation, and presentation of data (*statistical model*). Statistics, the discipline, has subdivisions, such as *biostatistics*, the application of statistical concepts and techniques to topics in the biomedical sciences. Statistics is also the **method** utilized in the discipline of statistics. Furthermore, statistics is the **collection of data through statistical methods**. Lastly, statistics can be **numbers that are computed from data in a sample**. Statistics from data in samples are represented by Latin letters and mathematical symbols; for example, $\bar{x}$ (x-bar) denotes a sample *mean*, and "s," "Std Dev," or "SD" denotes *standard deviation*. Data generated from or applied to a population are called *parameters*. Parameters are represented by Greek letters; for example, μ (mu) denotes the population mean and σ (sigma) signifies the population standard deviation.

Methods to summarize and analyze data in statistics are generally divided into two major categories—*descriptive statistics* and *inferential statistics* (Figure 1.1). Descriptive statistics (the category) is the analysis that helps describe and summarize statistics or parameters from samples and populations from which data have been collected. Examples of descriptive statistics (here statistics means data collected with statistical methods) include measures of *central tendency* (mean, *median*, or *mode*), measures of variability (e.g., standard deviation, range, *variance*), *distributions* of the data, and *confidence intervals*. As stated by Grimes and Schulz, "Descriptive studies often

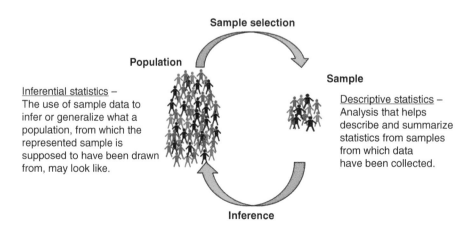

Figure 1.1 Descriptive and inferential statistics.

represent the first scientific toe in the water in new areas of inquiry. A fundamental element of descriptive reporting is a clear, specific, and measurable definition of the disease or condition in question. Like newspapers, good descriptive reporting answers the five basic W questions: who, what, why, when, where . . . and a sixth: so what?"[1] By itself, descriptive statistics cannot be used to form a conclusion about *associations* or intervention *effects* (e.g., a difference in disease status as a result of a treatment) and can therefore not answer a research hypothesis. Descriptive statistics does not infer, i.e., cannot induce, what the population from which a sample was drawn may look like.

As it is rarely feasible to collect data on a particular aspect of interest from everyone in a population, such as mean body weight of all men in New York City, a representative sample of men is drawn from the population of interest; from the statistics generated by this sample, we can use special statistical methods to estimate what the "true" (actual) mean weight might be if we had measured all men in the population (all men in New York City). The method used to estimate a parameter, differences between parameters, or associations between parameters based on sample statistics is called inferential statistics. In inferential statistics sample data are used to induce (infer, derive) what an unknown population parameter, from which the represented sample has been drawn, may look like—we basically extrapolate from the sample data to make an estimated induction about the population. It is even possible to make a claim for statistics being the science that tells whether something we observe can be generalized or applied to a new or different but similar situation. Obviously, inferential statistics is what we are mostly interested in to inform clinical care, and statistics (the discipline) helps us quantify the uncertainty or certainty of our generalizations and the probability of making an incorrect or correct conclusion.

It is important to realize that statistics can never provide absolute certainty. For example, if we want absolute certainty of what the mean body weight is among all adult men in New York City, we need to weigh each individual and then calculate the mean weight. If we could do this, we would have no use for inferential statistics. However, if we draw a representative sample from all men in New York City, we must take into consideration many uncertainties. With this in mind, statistics has been described as the "science of learning from data, and of measuring, controlling, and communicating uncertainty; and it thereby provides the navigation essential for controlling the course of scientific and societal advances."[2] One major goal of statistics is to enable decision making in the face of uncertainty. How and why these decisions are made form the basis for being an informed clinician.

Uncertainties can be reduced by utilizing specific statistical methods. For example, to get a representative sample of the population, we select men for our samples in a *randomized* manner; that is, every member of a population will have an equal chance of being selected into our sample. Nonrepresentative samples would, for example, be a selection of men who have gathered to participate in a sumo wrestling competition or those who are easily accessible to the researchers because they live nearby (i.e., *convenience sample*). Obviously, these men do not form a representative sample of all men in New York City. Another way to reduce uncertainty would be to select more rather than fewer men for our representative sample—increase the *sample size*. Assume there are approximately 3 million men in New York City—if we chose 10,000 instead of 10 men for our sample, there would be a greater chance that the mean weight calculated for the larger sample would better represent the true mean weight.

---

1 Grimes DA, Schulz KF. Descriptive studies: what they can and cannot do. *Lancet.* 2002; 359: 145–149.
2 Davidian M, Louis TA. Why statistics? *Science.* 2012; 6; 336(6077): 12.

Sampling is one of the most central and fundamental concepts underlying statistics. Accordingly, *random sampling error* or *random sampling variation* is an important concept to understand to correctly interpret scientific findings. Random sampling error is the name for differences or variations in characteristics of the sample and those of the general population from which the sample was drawn. Random sampling errors are always present and expected even in a random sampling process, as sample statistics can only approximate a population parameter. In other words, it is unlikely that sample characteristics, such as the mean body weight observed in a sample, will exactly reflect those of the population from where the sample was drawn, or that multiple samples from the same population will have the same mean weight. Another way of looking at sampling error is as an imperfect reflection of a parameter. Fortunately, there are statistical methods that can quantify this variation. The importance of variations in statistics is obvious when looking at the definition of statistics in the Medical Subject Headings (MeSH) thesaurus: "the science and art of collecting, summarizing, and analyzing data that are subject to random variation."

Methods used to compare samples or make probability predictions about data require *standardizing* or *normalizing* the data. Imagine a course in statistics where a student must take three quizzes and one final exam. The first quiz is worth 10%, the second 20%, and the third 30%, while the final exam is worth 40% of the course grade. Thus, if we consider a maximum of 100 points for a perfect grade in the course, the first quiz would account for a maximum of 10 points, the second quiz 20 points, the third quiz 30 points, and the final exam 40 points. If a student scored 90, 85, 70, and 95 on the quizzes and the final exam, respectively, what would be their final grade? One way to figure this out is to normalize the grades, that is, to calculate the "weight, or the contribution" of each grade to the total grade. The first quiz could have provided a maximum of 10 points, the second quiz 20 points, the third quiz 30 points, and the final exam 40 points. In the case of the student, the first quiz contributed 9 points (a score of 90% out of a possible 10 points), the second quiz 17 points (a score of 85% out of a possible 20 points), the third quiz 21 points (70% of 30), and the final exam 38 points (95% of 40), for a total of 85 out of a possible 100 points. The student's final grade would be 85. Although the student scored 90 on the first quiz and only 70 on the third quiz, the lower score on the third quiz contributed more to the final grade than the higher score on the first one. The described method normalized the exam scores by changing individual scores to a percentage of a total number of points. Essentially, the value of each score was converted from one unit (percentage of scores) to another unit (points). Normalizing, or standardizing, data is a key element utilized in statistical methods.

Beyond understanding what terms like *random* and errors represent in statistics, another often encountered term is distribution. A distribution is a representation of all possible values (or intervals) and the frequency (how often) of each value for a given *variable*. Such a distribution is often depicted graphically. Our example of mean body weight in a sample can be visualized by plotting each observed weight on the x-axis and the frequency—how often a specific weight is observed—on the y-axis (Figure 1.2). Each value can also be converted to a normalized score, such as a standard deviation (Figure 1.2). These normalized scores can also be represented as a distribution. There are different ways a distribution can be used. For example, one function of a distribution (a distribution function) can be used to calculate the probability of a variable's observed value.

The best known distribution and the most frequently encountered in statistical applications in the biomedical sciences is the *normal distribution*. The graphic depiction of a normal distribution (Figure 1.2) is often referred to as a bell curve or Gaussian curve. A normal distribution includes 100% of all possible scores, where 50% of the scores are above the mean (to the right of the mean) and 50% are below (to the left of the mean). Amazingly, when scores are normalized (converted) into units of standard deviations, 1 standard deviation above and 1 standard deviation below the

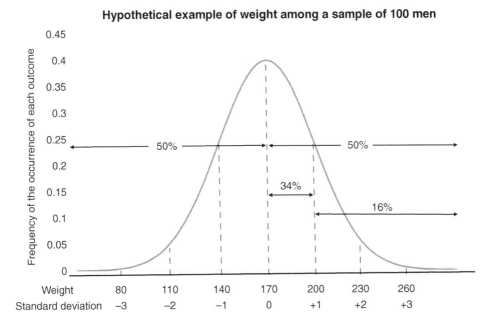

Figure 1.2   The Standard Normal Distribution.

mean always include approximately 68% of all possible scores (34% above and 34% below the mean); 2 standard deviations above and below the mean include a tad more than 95% of all possible scores; and 3 standard deviations above and below the mean include more than 99% of all possible scores (Figure 1.2). A standard deviation is the average difference between each collected score and the mean that we would expect from random samples of equal size drawn from the same population (Chapter 3).

Fundamental concepts throughout statistics are *precision* and *accuracy* (Figure 1.3). Precision is a function of replicability—how close to each other are replicated measurements—while accuracy is an estimation of how close the observed measurements are to the "truth" (the actual population parameter). Precision reflects *random errors* (variations among the values of a sample), while accuracy reflects *systematic errors* (errors that affect all values, due to, for example, inaccurate measurement tools, incorrect units, or other methodological flaws). Statistical methods can estimate both precision and accuracy, assisting in clinical decision making.

After data have been collected (gathering the data about the body weight of men in the sample), processed (entering the data into a format, e.g., a spreadsheet, to facilitate future tabulations), and explored (making appropriate measurements, such as frequency, mean, and variability), the data are analyzed for the final presentation of results. According to the Office of Research Integrity (ORI) at the U.S. Department of Health and Human Services, data analysis "is the process of systematically applying statistical and/or logical techniques to describe and illustrate, condense and recap, and evaluate data"[3] and "provide[s] a way of drawing inductive inferences from data and distinguishing the signal (the phenomenon of interest) from the noise (statistical fluctuations)

---

3 Office of Research Integrity, U.S. Department of Health and Human Services. Responsible conduct in data management. *Data Analysis* (https://ori.hhs.gov/education/products/n_illinois_u/datamanagement/datopic.html).

(a)   (b)

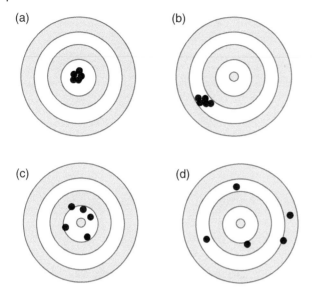

Figure 1.3 An analogy for precision and accuracy.
Interpretation of a shooter's precision and accuracy.
a) Precise and accurate
b) Precise but not accurate
c) Not precise but accurate
d) Not precise and not accurate

(c)   (d)

present in the data)."[4] Which statistical analysis is chosen is based on what the investigator wants to explore and the type of study.

Statistical techniques are applied never in a vacuum but in the context of a study design. Biomedical studies can broadly be divided into two major categories—*experimental studi*es, such as randomized controlled trials (Chapter 18), and *observational studies*, such as *cross-sectional studies*, *case-control studies*, and *cohort studies* (Chapters 15, 16, and 17). Designating a study as experimental or observational hinges on whether the investigator explicitly assigns an intervention or just observes a phenomenon without control of the administration of the intervention. For example, if an investigator wants to explore if a fluoride rinse (the intervention being studied) may reduce the *incidence* of caries, she may assign (i.e., select which study participants will and will not be assigned a fluoride mouth rinse) a fluoride mouth rinse to one group of study participants and a *placebo* rinse to another group of study participants, follow the participants for a specific period, and then compare the incidences of caries between the two groups. Another possibility is that the investigator could, instead of choosing to assign the intervention, enroll a group of individuals who are or have already been using a fluoride mouth rinse and compare the incidence of caries in this group to that in a group who are not or have not been using a fluoride mouth rinse. If the investigator assigned an intervention, the study is classified as an experimental study or a trial; if no intervention was assigned by the investigator, the study is classified as observational.

In general, most clinical studies assess frequencies of variables of interest, which form the basis for both descriptive and inferential statistics. Analyzing the body weight of men in New York City from a sample is one illustration of analyzing frequency data with the help of statistics. Another common and important concept is comparing frequency data between two or more samples or populations. Depending of what is being studied, comparisons can take place with an intervention (e.g., evaluate whether medication A is better than medication B, or measure if one dental implant causes more bone loss compared to another dental implant) or without an intervention. The former scenario occurs under the confines of an experimental or observational study and typically

---

4 Shamoo AE, Resnik BR. *Responsible Conduct of Research*. Oxford University Press; 2003.

compares the frequency of an outcome (a factor being predicted) to an *exposure* (any factor or characteristic that may explain or predict an outcome). The comparison can, after conducting analysis, be presented as an absolute comparison (e.g., *risk difference and mean difference*) or as a relative comparison (e.g., *risk ratio and odds ratio*). These comparisons are usually referred to as *measures of association* (Chapter 2).

Before an observed study result is published, it behooves the investigator to consider the *internal validity* (or simply *validity*) and the *external validity* (or *generalizability* or *applicability*) of the study. The internal validity is an assessment of whether or how bias and confounders and *random error* may have influenced the study outcome beyond the exposure. External validity is a measure of the generalizability of the study results.

Studies often report statistically significant or statistically nonsignificant findings. Unfortunately, the concept of statistical significance is often misunderstood and inappropriately reported. A good understanding and interpretation of statistical significance as well as recognizing the difference between statistical significance and clinical significance are essential to inform clinical practice. Several chapters in this book address these topics (Chapters 5, 6, 20).

One of the most important aspects for the reader of the biomedical literature is avoiding being misled by reported research results. This is a difficult task and entails being able to critically appraise the literature.[5] The following chapters arm the reader with important information on making informed clinical decisions, by providing a solid foundation for assessing the biomedical literature. However, it is beyond the scope of this book to highlight all possible misinterpretations and spins affecting the biomedical literature.[6]

Selected readings

Carrasco-Labra A, Brignardello-Petersen R, Glick M, Azarpazhooh A, Guyatt GH, eds. *How to Use Evidence-Based Dental Practices to Improve Your Clinical Decision Making.* ADA Publishing; 2020.

Carrasco-Labra A, Tampi M, Urquhart O, Howell S, Booth HA, Glick M. How to identify, interpret and apply the scientific literature to practice. In: Glick M, Greenberg MS, Lockhart PB, Challacombe S, eds. *Burket's Oral Medicine.* 13th ed. Wiley-Blackwell; 2021:1059–1079.

Cumming G. *Understanding the New Statistics: Effect Sizes, Confidence Intervals, and Meta-Analysis.* Routledge; 2012.

Glick M, Greenberg BL. A march toward scientific literacy. *J Am Dent Assoc.* 2017;148(8):543–545.

Greenberg BL, Glick M. Essential statistical and research design elements to help critically interpret the literature. In: Glick M, ed. *The Oral-Systemic Health Connection. A Guide to Patient Care.* 2nd ed. Quintessence; 2019: 24–37.

Hahs-Vaughn DL, Lomax RG. *An Introduction to Statistical Concepts.* 4th ed. Routledge; 2020.

Spiegelhalter DS. *The Art of Statistics: How to Learn from Data.* Basic Books; 2019.

Urdan TC. *Statistics in Plain English.* 5th ed. Routledge; 2022.

---

5 Carrasco-Labra A, Brignardello-Petersen R, Azarpazhooh A, Glick M, Guyatt GH. A practical approach to evidence-based dentistry: X: How to avoid being misled by clinical studies' results in dentistry. *J Am Dent Assoc.* 2015;146(12):919–924.

6 Boutron I, Ravaud P. Misinterpretation and distortion of research in biomedical literature. *PNAS.* 2018;115(11):2613–2619.

2

Understanding and interpreting measures of association

The primary aim of many *comparative effectiveness research* studies is to determine the impact of an *intervention* to inform clinical and policy decision making. The observed results of this type of research are often reported as estimates of the *magnitude* and direction of *effects* (i.e., desirable and undesirable consequences of applying an intervention are different directions of effects) that might be present in a *population*. In other words, researchers conduct a study of a *sample* from a population of interest to infer how big (the magnitude) of an effect can be anticipated in the population from which the sample was drawn and if the intervention improved or worsened (direction) a clinical *outcome*. Experiencing a clinical outcome is also sometimes referred to as having an *event*, and the terms are often used interchangeably.

Effect and effect size

An *effect size* is the size of the difference (i.e., subtraction) between two means usually expressed in units of standard deviation or as a ratio (i.e., division) between what is observed in a group of individuals who experienced an exposure (e.g., an *intervention or risk factor*) and what was observed in a *control group (comparison group)*—individuals who were not exposed to the intervention. Such a calculated difference or ratio is referred to as a *measure of association*. A control group may have been exposed to another known intervention or risk factor, a placebo, or nothing at all. Commonly used measures of association are absolute and relative measures of effect and can summarize the effect of interventions/exposures on outcomes that are measured both categorically (e.g., *dichotomous/binary variables*) and continuously. Absolute measures of association are depicted as the difference between effects in two groups. The most common absolute measures of effect include the *absolute risk difference* (ARD), which can be summed up as the *absolute risk reduction* (ARR) or *absolute risk increase* (ARI), and the *mean difference* (MD). Relative measures of association are depicted as the quotient of effects in two groups. The most common relative measures of effect include the *relative risk* (RR; note that RR may also be used for *risk ratio*, which is the same as relative risk) and can be summed up as the *relative risk difference* (RRD), also referred to as *relative risk reduction* (RRR) or *relative risk increase* (RRI), the *odds ratio* (OR), and the *ratio of means* (ROM).

Statistics for Dental Clinicians, First Edition. Michael Glick, Alonso Carrasco-Labra, and Olivia Urquhart.
© 2024 John Wiley & Sons, Inc. Published 2024 by John Wiley & Sons, Inc.

Dichotomous outcome variables

Consider the following example:

> In a hypothetical study to assess the association between smoking (exposure) and developing periodontal disease or not developing periodontal disease (a dichotomous outcome), a group of 1,000 individuals who smoke are followed for three years, and another group of 1,000 individuals, with the same risk factors for developing periodontal disease as the first group but who do not smoke, are also followed for three years. The observed results are as follows: 650 smokers developed periodontal disease, while only 150 nonsmokers did. The results are presented in Table 2.1.

Data presentation and interpretation

Absolute risk

In our hypothetical example, the *absolute risk* (AR) or probability for experiencing an event, or outcome (periodontal disease) among smokers (smoking is the "intervention" or "exposure"), is the total number of smokers with periodontal disease divided by the total number of individuals exposed to the intervention or risk factor (in this case smoking) over a three-year period. The AR for experiencing an event (periodontal disease) among nonsmokers is the total number of non-smokers with periodontal disease divided by the total number of individuals not exposed to the intervention or risk factor (in this case not smoking) over a three-year period. The AR can be expressed as a number ranging from 0 to 1 or as a percentage ranging from 0% to 100% Thus, we have an AR with the intervention and an AR without the intervention. The AR for developing

Table 2.1   Study outcome of a hypothetical study of developing periodontal disease among smokers and nonsmokers over a three-year time frame.

	Periodontal disease	No periodontal disease	No. of study participants
Smokers	650	350	1,000
Nonsmokers	150	850	1,000
	800	1,200	2,000

Absolute risk of developing periodontal disease among smokers equals 0.65 (Appendix 1, Equation 2.1a).
Absolute risk of developing periodontal disease among nonsmokers equals 0.15 (Appendix 1, Equation 2.1b).
Absolute risk reduction equals 0.50 (Appendix 1, Equation 2.2).
Relative risk of developing periodontal disease when smoking as compared with not smoking equals 4.33 (Appendix 1, Equation 2.3a).
Analogously, the relative risk of developing periodontal disease when not smoking as compared with smoking equals 0.23.
Relative risk difference equals 3.33 or 333% (Appendix 1, Equation 2.3b).
Odds of developing periodontal disease among smokers equals 1.86 (Appendix 1, Equation 2.4a).
Odds of developing periodontal disease among nonsmokers equals 0.18 (Appendix 1, Equation 2.4a).
Odds ratio for developing periodontal disease between smokers and nonsmokers equals 10.52 (Appendix 1, Equation 2.4b).
Odds of being a smoker among those with periodontal disease equals 4.33 (Appendix 1, Equation 2.5a).
Odds of being a smoker among those without periodontal disease equals 0.41 (Appendix 1, Equation 2.5a).
Odds ratio for being a smoker among those with and those without periodontal disease equals 10.52 (Appendix 1, Equation 2.5b).

periodontal disease among smokers was 65% but only 15% among nonsmokers (Table 2.1 and Appendix 1, Equations 2.1a, 2.1b).

Absolute risk difference

If we are interested in obtaining a single estimate that compares the AR of one group with that of another group, we calculate the ARR, ARI, or ARD. The ARD is an absolute measure of association and is the difference between the AR of developing periodontal disease among smokers compared to the AR of developing periodontal disease in nonsmokers. In our hypothetical example, as smoking was associated with an AR of developing periodontal disease of 65% in smokers and 15% in nonsmokers, the ARD was 50 percentage points (Table 2.1 and Appendix 1, Equation 2.2).

In plain English, based on our observed data (Table 2.1) we can state the following:

- Smoking is associated with an AR (chance, *probability*) for developing periodontal disease of 65% after three years.
- After three years, 65% of smokers can expect to develop periodontal disease.
- Not smoking is associated with an AR (chance, probability) for developing periodontal disease of 15% after three years.
- After three years, 15% of nonsmokers can expect to develop periodontal disease.
- As 65% of smokers were expected to develop periodontal disease and 15% of nonsmokers were expected to develop periodontal disease over a period of 3 years, the attribution of smoking for developing periodontal disease is 50%.

Relative risk or risk ratio

Relative risks compare the AR of an event occurring (in our example periodontal disease), after an *exposure* (in our example smoking) with an event occurring (periodontal disease), in a comparison group (*control group* or reference group) that has not experienced the exposure (in our example not smoking). The RR is a relative measure of association and is expressed as a quotient (i.e., division) of the AR in one group and the AR in the other group, without any units. In our example (Table 2.1), the RR for developing periodontal disease when smoking compared to not smoking was 4.33 and the RRD is 333% (Table 2.1 and Appendix 1, Equations 2.3a, 2.3b). Analogously, the RR for developing periodontal disease when not smoking compared to smoking was 0.23 (23%) and the RRD is −77% (23% − 100% = − 77%).

In plain English, based on our observed data (Table 2.1) we can state the following:

- The risk of developing periodontal disease among smokers is 4.33 that of nonsmokers after three years.
- Smoking relative to not smoking for three years is associated with 3.33 times greater or 333% greater risk of developing periodontal disease.
- The risk of developing periodontal disease among nonsmokers is 0.23, or 23%, that of smokers after three years.
- Not smoking relative to smoking for three years is associated with a 77% decreased risk of developing periodontal disease.

Describing the increased or decreased risk of an outcome occurring as *that of* and *greater than* may seem confusing but is an important distinction when interpreting study results. Using a more familiar example may help the clarify the difference of such sentence structure. If person A has $120 and person B has $100, person A has 1.2 times *that of* person B, or person A has 0.20 or 20%

more money than person B. Analogously, if person B has $100 and person C has $80, person C has 0.80 or 80% *that of* person B, or person C has 20% *less* money than person B.

Odds ratio

The AR discussed above is a probability—an event occurring as a proportion of all possible events. In contrast, the *odds* represent the likelihood of an event occurring as a proportion of the event not occurring. For example, the probability of throwing a 6 with one 6-sided die is

$$\frac{an\ event\ (throwing\ a\ 6)}{all\ possible\ events\ (1,2,3,4,5,and\ 6)} = \frac{1}{6}, \text{ or } 0.17, \text{ while the odds of throwing a 6 with one 6-sided die}$$

is $\dfrac{\dfrac{an\ event\ (throwing\ a\ 6)}{all\ possible\ events\ (1,2,3,4,5,and\ 6)}}{\dfrac{an\ event\ not\ occurring\ (throwing\ a\ 1,2,3,4,and\ 5)}{all\ possible\ events\ (1,2,3,4,5,and\ 6)}}, \dfrac{\dfrac{1}{6}}{\dfrac{5}{6}} = \dfrac{1}{5},$ or 0.20. An OR measures the relative

strength of an association between an outcome and an *exposure*, where the odds (the likelihood) of an event occurring are compared to the odds (the likelihood) of it not occurring between the groups under comparison (the odds in the intervention group compared to the odds in the reference group), or vice versa. In our hypothetical example (Table 2.1), the OR may thus reflect the likelihood of developing periodontal disease or not between smokers and nonsmokers, but it could also reflect the likelihood of smoking or not smoking between someone who has periodontal disease and someone who does not. The odds of developing periodontal disease in our example among smokers are 1.86, and the odds of developing periodontal disease among nonsmokers are 0.18 (Table 2.1 and Appendix 1, Equation 2.4a), which result in an OR of 10.52 (Table 2.1 and Appendix 1, Equation 2.4b, 2.5b).

In plain English, based on our observed data (Table 2.1) we can state the following:

- For every 1.86 persons developing periodontal disease when smoking, 1 person will not develop periodontal disease when smoking, or for every 186 persons developing periodontal disease when smoking, 100 persons will not develop periodontal disease when smoking.
- For every 0.18 persons developing periodontal disease when not smoking, 1 person will not develop periodontal disease when smoking, or for every 18 persons developing periodontal disease when not smoking, 100 persons will not develop periodontal disease when smoking.
- The odds for every 10.52 persons developing periodontal disease when smoking, 1 person has an odds to develop periodontal disease when not smoking, or the odds for every 1,052 persons developing periodontal disease when smoking, 100 persons have an odds to develop periodontal disease when not smoking.

Mean difference

Consider a hypothetical example:

> A hypothetical study assesses the effect of scaling and root planning compared to no scaling or root planning on clinical attachment loss (CAL) after three months of follow-up. The *average* CAL values were 1.5 mm in the scaling and root planning group and 3.5 mm in the no treatment group. The previous example of developing periodontal disease involved a dichotomous variable. In contrast, measurements of CAL are *continuous variables*.

The difference in CAL between the two groups is –2.0 mm (Appendix 1, Equation 2.6). This is an absolute measure of association called a *mean difference* (MD)—a difference between two means. A negative number suggests that the intervention group has a lower mean score on an outcome compared to the control group, whereas a positive number indicates a higher mean score. In plain English, an MD of –2.0 mm in our example suggest that on average individuals who underwent scaling and root planning had a CAL of 2.0 mm less than the control group.

A few additional notes

- Absolute risk represents an *incidence* (number of people developing a condition during a specific time interval).
- Incidence can be expressed as an *incidence proportion*—the number of disease-free people at baseline who experience an event as a proportion of the total number of people who are eligible to experience the event at baseline—or as an *incidence rate*—the number of disease-free people at baseline who experience an event as a proportion of the time all people who are eligible to experience the event contributed to the study period.
- *Risk* in statistics is not only a measure of harm but can also be interpreted as benefit. Put another way, risk in statistical terms expresses the probability, or the chance, that an event will occur, without any judgment as to whether the outcome is beneficial (Chapter 1). By convention, when calculating an RR the risk of experiencing an outcome in the intervention group is usually placed in the numerator and the risk of developing an outcome in the nonintervention group is placed in the denominator. Thus, an RR > 1 suggests that the risk is greater for an event among persons receiving the intervention or having an exposure, compared to the risk of an event among those not receiving the intervention or experiencing the exposure. An RR < 1 suggests that the risk for an event is reduced among persons receiving the intervention or having an exposure, compared to the risk among those not exposed. An RR = 1 suggests that there is no difference in experiencing an event between those receiving the intervention or experiencing the exposure (Table 2.2). In our example (Table 2.1), the RR of developing periodontal disease when smoking compared to not smoking was 4.33, but the RR of developing periodontal disease when not smoking (not smoking is now the intervention of interest) compared to smoking (the control or reference group) was 0.23 (23%), or a reduction of 0.77 (77%) (Table 2.1).
- Similar to RR, an OR > 1 is associated with higher odds of the outcome given the exposure compared to the reference group, an OR < 1 is associated with lower odds of the outcome given the exposure compared to the reference group, and an OR = 1 is interpreted as no difference in the outcome given the exposure compared to the reference group. Also, an OR of 1.86 means there is an 86% increase and an OR of 3 indicates a 200% increase in the odds of an outcome with a given exposure compared to the reference group. Although an OR of 3 is a tripling of the *odds* of the outcome, this is not the same as a tripling of the *risk* (Figure 2.1).
- The *number needed to treat for benefit (NNTB)* and the *number needed to treat for harm (NNTH)* are two other related measures of association encountered in the medical literature. Both are calculated by taking the inverse of the ARD. The NNTB is defined as the number of individuals in the intervention group who would need to be treated for one person to experience a positive outcome, whereas the NNTH represents the number of individuals in the intervention group who need to be treated for one person to avoid a harmful outcome.

Table 2.2 Interpretation of relative risk and odds ratio in different study designs.

	Relative Risk	Odds Ratio
Experimental studies		
Randomized trial (for comparing treatments or interventions)	The risk of developing disease among those who are exposed relative to the risk of developing disease among those who are not exposed; the ratio of the incidence of new disease among the exposed relative to the nonexposed; an RR >1 suggest the exposure is a risk factor for developing the disease; a RR <1 suggests an exposure is protective against developing the disease; a RR = 1 suggests there is no association between the exposure and disease.	The odds that an exposed person develops disease relative to the odds that a nonexposed person develops disease; an OR >1 suggests the exposure is positively associated the disease; an OR <1 suggests the exposure is negatively associated with the disease; an OR = 1 suggests no association between exposure and disease.
Observational studies		
Cohort study	The risk of developing disease among those who are exposed relative to the risk of developing disease among those who are not exposed; the ratio of the incidence of new disease among the exposed relative to the nonexposed; an RR >1 suggest the exposure is a risk factor for developing the disease; a RR <1 suggests an exposure is protective against developing the disease; a RR = 1 suggests there is no association between the exposure and disease.	The odds that an exposed person develops disease relative to the odds that a nonexposed person develops disease; an OR >1 suggests the exposure is positively associated the disease; an OR <1 suggests the exposure is negatively associated with the disease; an OR = 1 suggests no association between exposure and disease.
Case-control study	Cannot be calculated directly	The odds of those with disease having been exposed relative to the odds of those without disease having been exposed; an OR >1 suggests the exposure is positively associated with the exposure; an OR <1 suggests the exposure is negatively associated with the disease; an OR = 1 suggests no association.
Cross-sectional study	Cannot be calculated	Cannot be calculated unless there is a comparison group; in that case similar to interpretation for a case-control study.
Case report/case series	Cannot be calculated	Cannot be calculated

Glick M, Greenberg BL. Primer to biostatistics for busy clinicians. In: Carrasco-Labra A, Brignardello-Petersen A, Glick M, Azarpazooh A, Guyatt G, eds. *How to Use Evidence-Based Dental Practice to Improve Your Clinical Decision-Making.* American Dental Association Publishing; 2020:185–208.

	CVD(+)	CVD(−)	Absolute risk of CVD(+) if PD(+)	Absolute risk of CVD(+) if PD(−)	Odds of CVD(+) if PD(+)	Odds of CVD(+) if PD(−)
PD(+)	50	50	50/100 = 0.5		50/50 = 1	
PD(−)	25	75		25/100 = 0.25		25/75 = 1/3

Figure 2.1 Hypothetical study results showing that an odds ratio can be very different from a risk ratio. The odds of CVD(+) given PD(+) compared with the odds of CVD(+) given PD(−) is 3:1. Thus, an odds ratio 3. However, the risk of CVD(+) given PD(+) compared with the risk of CVD(+) given PD(−) is 2:1. Thus, a risk ratio of 2. CVD(+) – presence of cardiovascular disease; CVD(−) – absence of cardiovascular disease; PD(+) – presence of periodontal disease; PD(−) – absence of periodontal disease.

- All measures of association discussed (RR, OR, ARD, MD) are point estimates that have more clinical relevance when accompanied by a *confidence interval* (Chapters 6 and 20). Thus, confidence intervals should also be reported in conjunction with respective measures of association.
- Estimates of RR and OR are usually similar when the event being assessed is rare or has a frequency below 10% to 15%. However, substantial differences between RR and OR are evident when assessing more common events.
- When assessing clinical relevance (Chapter 20), RRs and ORs should always be judged in the context of *baseline risk*. For example, if, hypothetically, we found that using glucocorticosteroids (GCS) for the treatment of lichen planus is associated with the development of oropharyngeal cancer (OPC) with an RR of 6, we can state that using GCS is associated with a sixfold risk of developing OPC. However, if we assume that in the age group we are studying the baseline risk of OPC is 0.02%, the sixfold risk would result in an incidence of 0.12% (6 × 0.02%). At an individual level, this risk is very small and probably clinically irrelevant.
- An interpretation of an OR is a complicated and difficult concept to explain to patients. Furthermore, an OR from a study may often be based on an incidence that is different than that in the population. For example, when studying a disease with a low incidence, researchers may have to include a larger proportion of cases in their study than that in a population. For these reasons, there may be a need to convert an OR to a RR (Table 2.3 and Appendix 1, Formula 2.10).

Table 2.3 Equating on odds ratio to a relative risk as a function of different incidences in an unexposed population.

		Incidence		
		0.1	0.3	0.5
Odds ratio	1.5	1.43	1.30	1.20
	2.0	1.82	1.54	1.33
	2.5	2.17	1.72	1.43
	3.0	2.50	1.88	1.50
	3.5	2.80	2.00	1.56
	4.0	3.08	2.11	1.60

For example, an odds ratio of 3.0 equates to a relative risk of 1.88 in a population with an incidence of 0.3 (Appendix 1, Formula 2.10, Figure 2.2).

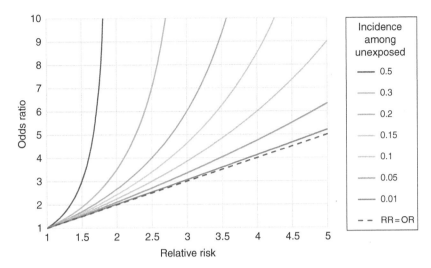

Figure 2.2 Equating an odds ratio to a relative risk as a function of the incidence among unexposed.

As evident in this Table 2.3 and Figure 2.2, different incidences may create important differences between an RR derived from an OR in a study and an RR derived from the same study but used in a different patient population.

An application of measures of association to retail

You want to tell a friend about the purchase of a discounted jacket. Instead of the original price of $80, you paid only $32. How are you going to convince her to buy the same jacket? There are different ways you can frame your purchase:

- The sale price of the jacket was only $32.
- The price of the jacket was only 40% of the original price.
- I got a 60% discount.
- I got a $48 discount.

"The sale price of the jacket was only $32." The sale price is the difference between the original price and the sale discount (all in dollars)−$80 − $48 = $32. This is analogous to the absolute risk with the intervention.

"The price of the jacket was only 40% that of the original price." The sale price as a percentage of the original (baseline) cost−$32 / $80 = 0.40−is 40%. This is analogous to after an intervention (absolute risk with the intervention) divided by the baseline risk (absolute risk without the intervention), which equals the relative risk (RR).

"I got a 60% discount." The sale discount is the difference between the original price and the discounted price (in percentages). As these prices are in percentages, the original price equals 100%, the sale price equals 40%, and the sale discount equals 60%. This is analogous to the relative risk difference.

"I got a $48 discount." The sale discount is the difference between the original price (absolute risk without the intervention) and the sale price (absolute risk with the intervention) (all in dollars)—$80 – $32 = $48. This is analogous to the absolute risk reduction (ARR) or absolute risk difference (ARD).

Returning to the issue of *that of* and *greater than*, with our retail example we can state that $80 is 2.5 times or 250% that of $32, but we can also state that $80 is 150% more than $32.

Let's examine a second example. A jacket originally priced $800 is on sale for $320 (40% that of the original price). Although the sale price as a percentage of the original cost is the same as in the previous example—the equivalent of an RR of 0.40 in both examples—there is a difference in how much we paid for the jacket ($32 vs. $320).

What are you most interested in—a sale price as a percentage of the original price (RR = 40%) or how much money you are willing to spend on the jacket ($32 or $320) (absolute risk with the intervention)? Obviously, depending on how much money you have, the sale price as a percentage of the original price (RR) needs to be viewed within the context of the original price (baseline risk). This is equivalent to insisting that an RR needs to be assessed within the context of absolute risk without the intervention.

Selected readings

Andrade C. Understanding relative risk, odds ratio, and related terms: as simple as it can get. *J Clin Psychiatry.* 2015;76(7):e857–e861.

Cumming G. *Understanding the New Statistics: Effect Sizes, Confidence Intervals, and Meta-Analysis.* Routledge; 2012.

Monaghan TF, Rahman SN, Agudelo CW, et al. Foundational statistical principles in medical research: a tutorial on odds ratios, relative risk, absolute risk, and number to treat. *Int J Environ Res Public Health.* 2021;18(11):5669. https://doi.org/10.3390/ijerph18115669.

Norton EC, Dowd BE, Maciejewski ML. Odds ratios—current best practice. *J Am Med Assoc.* 2018;320(1):84–85.

Sedgwick P. Absolute and relative risks. *BMJ.* 2012;345:e5613.

Sedgwick P. What are odds? *BMJ.* 2012;344:e2853.

Sedgwick P. What are the odds? *BMJ.* 2015;350:h2327.

Sedgwick P. What are the risks? *BMJ.* 2015;345:e2853.

3

Understanding and interpreting a standard deviation and normal distribution

When presenting quantitative data, we provide meaningful measures that can be easily understood and used to interpret the data. Clinical research often utilizes *randomly* drawn samples from a population of interest. Randomly selected means that every individual in a sample has an equal chance of being selected, while a *sample* is a representative group selected from a *population*. In statistical terms a population represents the whole group for which results are applicable, or a group about which we want to draw a conclusion. For example, if we want information about the weight of all men in New York City (NYC), it would not be feasible to individually weigh each one. So instead we choose to randomly select 100 men, calculate their *mean* weight (the arithmetic average), and then infer from this sample what the mean weight is among the whole population of men in NYC. The sample mean provides a description of one measure that could be useful, but our data may offer even more information that could help derive information, such as the *probability* of finding a man above or below a particular weight or a range of weights, and much more. One measure that is often used to infer or describe continuous data of a population is the *standard deviation*. "Deviation" in statistical terms refers to variation, variability, *spread*, or dispersion, while "standard" denotes typical or average. In short, standard deviation is a measure of the average dispersion of values around a mean we would expect from random samples of equal size drawn from the same population.

Imagine that in one randomly drawn sample of 100 men the average body weight is 170 lbs., with the weights equally distributed between 140 and 200 lbs. In another random sample of 100 men the average weight is also 170 lbs., with the weights equally distributed between 110 lbs. and 230 lbs. By looking only at the mean, one can infer that there is no difference between the samples. However, the weights in the first example are more bunched together (have less variability, are less dispersed)—with a range of 60 lbs. (200 lbs. − 140 lbs. = 60 lbs.)—than compared with the second sample where the weights are more dispersed (larger variability) around the mean—with a range of 120 lbs. (230 lbs. − 110 lbs. = 120 lbs.). The first sample has a smaller standard deviation compared with the second sample.

A collection of all scores on a *variable* (a variable is anything that can be codified and has more than one value; in our example the variable is weight) is often referred to as a *distribution* of scores. A common distribution to describe continuous data is the *normal distribution*, often described as a bell curve (Figure 3.1a). In the graph of a normal distribution the scores are displayed on the x-axis, while the frequency of the occurrence of a score is shown on the y-axis. As can be appreciated, when looking at this curve the most frequent scores correspond with the middle of the scores on the x-axis—where the middle represents a mean, or a *median*, score. Another realization is how

Statistics for Dental Clinicians, First Edition. Michael Glick, Alonso Carrasco-Labra, and Olivia Urquhart.
© 2024 John Wiley & Sons, Inc. Published 2024 by John Wiley & Sons, Inc.

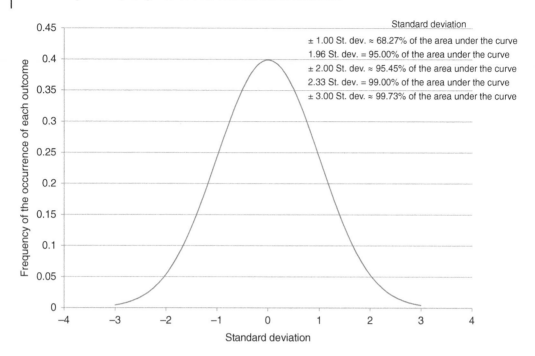

Figure 3.1a Standard normal distribution.

the graph of the normal distribution displays extreme values (in our case, very light and very heavy men) as rare (least frequent), displayed at the tail ends of the curve.

A normal distribution includes 100% of all possible scores where 50% of the scores are above the mean and 50% of the scores are below the mean. One standard deviation surrounding the mean always includes approximately 68% (or more exact 68.268949%) of all possible scores (Figure 3.1b); 2 standard deviations surrounding the mean always include a tad more than 95% (or more exact 95.449974%) of all possible scores (Figure 3.1c); and 3 standard deviations surrounding the mean always include more than 99% (or more exact 99.730020%) of all possible scores (Figure 3.1d).

A percentage, for example 68%, is the percentage of the total area that can be found under the curve between −1 standard deviation and +1 standard deviation (Figure 3.1b) and equals the percentage of scores within this area.

As one standard deviation surrounding the mean includes approximately 68% of all possible scores and the scores are symmetrically distributed around the mean, 34% of all scores are below and 34% scores are above the mean (Figure 3.2).

In our hypothetical example of a sample of 100 men whose body weight follows a normal distribution (Figure 3.2), their mean body weight is 170 lbs., with a calculated standard deviation of 30 lbs. Of the men, 50% weigh *below* and 50% weigh *above* 170 lbs. In addition, we know that 34.13% of men weigh *between* 170 and 200 lbs. (the mean + 1 standard deviation [170 lbs. + 30 lbs. = 200 lbs.]) and 34.13% weigh *between* 170 lbs. and 140 lbs. (the mean − 1 standard deviation [170 lbs. − 30 lbs. = 140 lbs.]). Also, 84.13% (the mean + 1 standard deviation [50% + 34.13% = 84.13%]) weigh *less* than 200 lbs., and therefore the remaining 15.87% of men weigh *above* 200 lbs. Consistent with the above argument, we can state that if we randomly select a man from our population, there is an 84.13% chance (probability) of him weighing below 200 lbs. and a 15.87% chance of him weighing above 200 lbs.

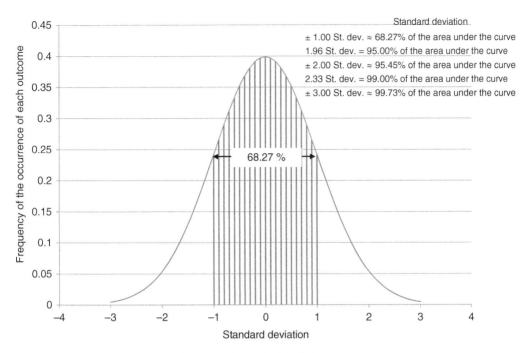

Figure 3.1b Standard normal distribution—±1 standard deviation.

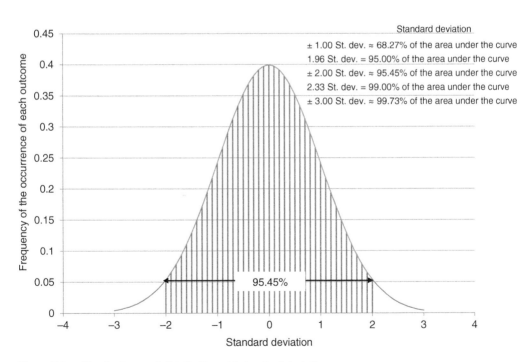

Figure 3.1c Standard normal distribution—±2 standard deviations.

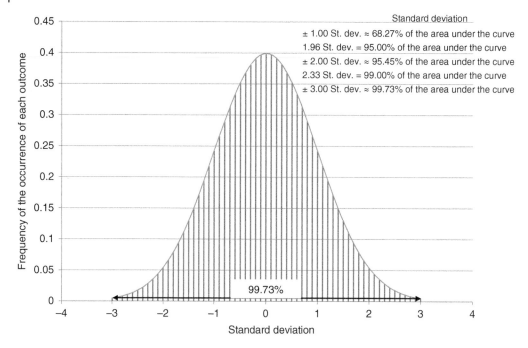

Figure 3.1d   Standard normal distribution−±3 standard deviations.

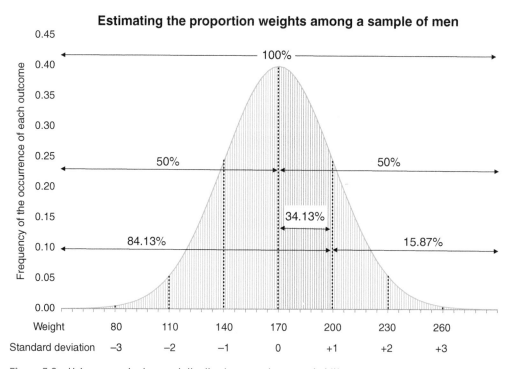

Figure 3.2   Using a standard normal distribution to estimate probability.

Essentially, what we have done is converted (*standardized*) our scores (the values, or scores, of weights) into another unit (a standard deviation unit) that can be used to estimate another *metric*, or measurement—the area under the curve. Converting a score into a standard deviation unit of measurement enables us not only to compare samples but also to estimate probabilities. We do this by calculating an individual score expressed as a difference from the mean in a standard deviation unit. Such a standard deviation unit is called the *z-score*—the total number of deviations of any given data point that lies above or below the mean and is the quotient of the difference between a score and the mean, and the standard deviation (Appendix 1, Formula 3.1a, 3.1b). A z-score below the mean is denoted with a minus sign, one above the mean with a plus sign (Figure 3.3). A z-score table (Appendix 2. Z-table) will display the total area under the curve to the left of a particular score. For example, looking at the table, a z-score of +1.00 equals 0.8413. Thus, the area under the curve from +1.00 standard deviations above the mean to the beginning of the curve is 0.8413, or 84.13%. In our example (Figure 3.2), there is an 84.13% chance of finding a man with a weight less than 200 lbs. Again, looking at the table, there is a 50.00% chance of finding a man below 170 lbs., which means there is a 34.13% probability (84.13% − 50.00% = 34.13%) of finding a man with a weight between 170 and 200 lbs.

Any random sample of weights drawn from a population has a normal distribution. Such a distribution displayed with standard deviations where the mean equals 0 standard deviations and each score is displayed according to its distance from the mean in a unit of standard deviations is called a *standard normal distribution* (Figures 3.1, 3.2, and 3.3). As in our example, if the mean weight of a drawn sample is 170 lbs. with a standard deviation of 30 lbs., the score of 170 lbs. is represented by a standard deviation of 0 and a score of 200 lbs. is represented by +1 standard deviation (170 lbs. + 30 lbs. = 200 lbs.) (Figure 3.2).

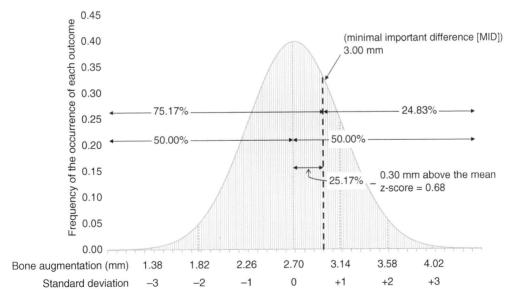

Figure 3.3   Hypothetical example of bone augmentation.

Consider a hypothetical example:

> A clinician wants to know the amount of bone generated after using a bone graft when placing a dental implant. The clinician selected at random 20 individuals from her population of 400 patients who have received a bone graft after the placement of a single anterior implant and reviewed their records. Six months after placing the bone graft, she examined how much bone had been generated around the implant. Her data revealed a mean bone augmentation of 2.70 mm with a calculated standard deviation of 0.44 (mean bone augmentation 2.70 ± 0.44 mm).

What does this really mean?

She had previously determined that a bone increase of 3.00 mm or more would be clinically significant and important to patients (i.e., long-term implant stability, cost of the procedure to attain this level of bone augmentation, physical and emotional burden associated with the procedure, and other patient-important outcomes). This level is also known as the *minimal important difference* (MID) (Chapter 20).

Using the argument on how to estimate the probability above, the standard deviation can also help to estimate the probability of achieving more or less bone augmentation. As we saw before, using specific formulas (Appendix 1, Formula 3.1) including the sample mean and standard deviation, it is possible to convert every score (millimeters of increased bone) into a standard deviation unit, a z-score, and calculate a probability of attaining any particular score. For example, the chance of attaining 3.0 mm or less bone equals a probability of 75.17% (Equation 3.1) and the chance of generating 0.30 mm more bone than the mean is 25.17% (Figure 3.3).

A few additional notes

- A normal distribution is asymptotic, which mean the tails of the curve come very close to but never reach 0 on the x-axis.
- A standard deviation of a sample is sometimes abbreviated as *s* or sd.
- A standard deviation of a population can be abbreviated as σ (sigma).
- The standard deviation is used to estimate statistical data, such as probabilities, confidence intervals, *standard error*, and more.
- Standard deviation is a statistic that describes variability in a sample and is not the same as standard error, which is an inferential statistic that estimates the variability of several samples to infer what a distribution of means would look like (Chapter 4).
- Standard deviation can be calculated from sample means (Appendix 1, Formula 3.2), sample proportions (Appendix 1, Formula 3.3), and more.
- Formulas for standard deviation are identical to those for standard error, except that standard deviation formulas use statistics whereas standard error equations use parameters.

An application of standardization to estimate the volume of a bowl

We have been tasked with estimating the volume of a bowl. This might sound like a complicated mathematical exercise, but we can simplify this task. We construct a square container that can hold exactly 1 liter of water. The volume of this container can be calculated without too much difficulty (height × width × length). Thus, we now know the volume of 1 liter of water.

Now we fill our bowl with water. The amount of water, as measured by how many liters are used to fill the bowl, can now be converted to volume as we know the volume of 1 liter. We have essentially converted the unit of volume to another unit of measurement. This is what we do when we convert a score (a measurement) in one unit (e.g., millimeters) to a unit of standard deviation.

We can take this one step further and compare the volume of different shapes of containers, such as bowls, ewers, flasks, and so on, using our new standardized measure, the quantity of water as measured by liters.

Selected readings

Sedgwick P. Normal distribution. *BMJ.* 2012;345:e6533.
Sedgwick P. Standard deviation or the standard error of the mean. *BMJ.* 2015;350:h831.

4

Understanding and interpreting standard error

One of the most important aspects of statistics is the ability to make inferences about a *population* based on a *sample* drawn from the population. In statistical terms we want to use a sample *statistic* to estimate a population *parameter*. This type of statistics is referred to as *inferential statistics*, and the *standard error* (SE) is used to estimate the precision of our inferences.

Feasibility and resource constraints prevent researchers from examining every member of a population, such as all men in New York City (NYC). This is where statistics come to help, allowing researchers to estimate, based on a representative sample (a representative individual or group) drawn from a specific *target population* (all members of the group about which we want to make a conclusion, the population of interest), what the entire population might look like.

Inferential statistics is the branch of statistics used to derive (infer, generalize) characteristics of an entire population based on a sample drawn from said population. For example—using inferential statistical methods—based on a calculated mean of a single sample (e.g., the mean height of a sample of men in NYC), it is possible to estimate, with some degree of precision, the difference compared with any other sample mean drawn, using the same methods, from this population, and the difference between the drawn sample and the actual population mean. This information is very helpful, as it is highly likely that if we draw several samples of the same size from the same population, every sample will have a different mean. A compilation of all these hypothetical sample means is often referred to as the *sampling distribution* of the mean. A *distribution* in statistics refers to a collection of all scores in a sample.

Fortunately, it is sufficient to look at only a single sample mean to estimate how other sample means—if drawn from the same population using identical methodology—might differ from the actual population mean. To do this, the SE is used. When the SE is used with means, it is called the *standard error of the mean* (SEM), but there are also other standard error measurements, such as the *standard error of a sample proportion*. For the sake of simplicity, a sample mean and SEM are used throughout this chapter as an example of SE. The main idea behind using SE is to estimate *sampling error*, or how far the calculated sample mean is from the actual population mean. A smaller SE as opposed to a larger SE suggests the sample mean is closer to the actual population mean (Figure 4.1). The formula for SE includes the sample size in the denominator (Formula 4.1). Thus, the larger the sample size, the smaller the SE. The standard error provides an estimate of how precise the sample mean is. This precision is often expressed as a *confidence interval* (CI) (Chapter 6), which is estimated using a formula that includes SE (Formula 4.2).

Consider the following example.

A clinician has been encouraged to measure her patients' systolic blood pressure (SBP) before performing an extraction. As some of her patients may have a raised SBP, she might consider advising them to use a blood-pressure-lowering medication. She decides to perform a study to ascertain what the SBP might be among asymptomatic patients, without a history of hypertension (HTN),

Statistics for Dental Clinicians, First Edition. Michael Glick, Alonso Carrasco-Labra, and Olivia Urquhart.

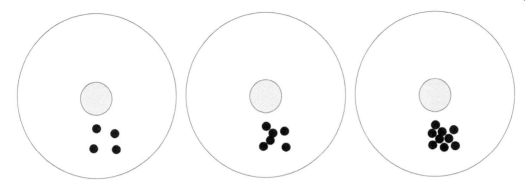

Figure 4.1 Relationship between sample size and standard error. The more shots with the same gun, from the same position and by the same shooter, will provide better and better precision (tighter cluster of shots). This is similar to increasing the sample size in a study, which will decrease the standard error (Formula 4.1). A lower standard error provides a more narrow confidence interval and better precision.

who either receive a blood-pressure-lowering drug or do not. After acquiring all the necessary permission to perform this study, she gathers the data according to an acceptable methodology.

From her total patient population, she selects 20 patients who are asymptomatic, do not have a history of HTN, and do not take any blood-pressure-lowering medications and divides them into two groups. Group 1 consists of 10 patients who will not receive the blood-pressure-lowering medication, and group 2 consists of 10 patients who will receive the medication. She measures and records the SBP of all 20 patients.

The result from group 1 is as follows: the SBP values range from a low of 110 mm Hg to a high of 140 mm Hg; the mean SBP is 122.90 mm Hg; and the SD is 8.76 mm Hg, which can be written as mean (SD) = 122.90 mm Hg (8.76 mm Hg) (Chapter 3). The result from group 2 is as follows: the SBP values range from a low of 103 mm Hg to a high of 130 mm Hg; mean (SD) = 113.80 mm Hg (10.05 mm Hg).

As the clinician is interested in using her data to infer what she could expect to find among all her asymptomatic patients without a history of HTN, she calculates the SEM (Appendix 1, Equation 4.1) and then is able to calculate a 95% CI for both groups (Appendix 1, Equation 4.2) (Chapter 6). For group 1 the SEM is 2.77 and the 95% CI has a range from 117.47 mm Hg to 128.33 mm Hg. This can be written as mean (SEM) = 122.90 mm Hg (2.77 mm Hg); and mean (95% CI) = 122.90 mm Hg (95% CI; 117.47 mm Hg to 128.33 mm Hg). For group 2, mean (SEM) = 113.80 mm Hg (3.18 mm Hg); and mean (95% CI) = 113.80 mm Hg (95% CI; 107.57 mm Hg to 120.03 mm Hg).

Interpretation of the standard error of the mean

As 1 SEM for group 1 was 2.77 mm Hg, 2 SEM is 5.54 mm Hg (2 × 2.77 mm Hg = 5.54 mm Hg); and as 1 SEM in group 2 was 3.18 mm Hg, 2 SEM in group 2 is 6.36 mm Hg (2 × 3.18 = 6.36 mm Hg). Thus, she can expect that 95% (≈2 SEM) (Chapter 3)[1] of all her asymptomatic patients without a history of HTN who will not receive any blood-pressure-lowering medication would be within ±5.54 mm Hg from the actual mean of asymptomatic patients without a history of HTN patients in her patient population who do not receive blood-pressure-lowering medications (group 1); and she can expect

---

1 In a normal standard distribution, a 95% confidence interval surrounds a mean by ±1.96 SEM or standard deviations, but we can use 2 SEM as an approximation.

that 95% ($\approx$2 SEM) of patients who receive blood-pressure-lowering medications would be within $\pm$6.36 mm Hg from the actual mean of her patient population who do not receive blood-pressure-lowering medications (group 2) (recall that she selected all her patients in her study from a group of asymptomatic patients without a history of HTN who did not take any blood-pressure-lowering medications).

Implication of the standard error of the mean

She can now state that even if she didn't measure the SBP in all her asymptomatic patients without a history of HTN who didn't take any blood-pressure-lowering medications, she is 95% confident that her patients have an SBP of between 117 mm Hg and 128 mm Hg (rounded to whole numbers) even if they hadn't received a blood pressure medication; and she is also 95% confident that even if she didn't measure the SBP in all her asymptomatic patients without a history of HTN who didn't take any blood-pressure-lowering medications and who were given the blood-pressure-lowering medication, they would have an SBP between 108 mm Hg and 120 mm Hg (rounded to whole numbers).

From a clinical perspective she would be concerned with treating a patient with an SBP above 130 mm Hg. Thus, if she had administered or not administered blood-pressure-lowering medications to every asymptomatic patient with no history of HTN who didn't take any blood-pressure-lowering medications, the results would not have been clinically important since in both groups the chance of having an SBP above 130 is very small (i.e., 130 is outside of the range of the 95% confidence intervals for both groups).

Standard errors can also be used to determine statistical significance of differences of means. In our example the difference of the means was 9.1 mm Hg with a SD of 8.76 mm Hg for group 1 and a SD of 10.05 mm Hg for group 2. These values will provide a p-value of 0.04, which, with a significance level of <0.05, is a statistically significant finding (Chapter 5) (Appendix 1, Equation 4.3 and Appendix 3).

A few additional notes

- There are similarities and differences between *standard deviation* and standard error.

  A sample randomly drawn from a population of interest is but one of many possible samples that could have been drawn. Each sample would probably not have the same characteristics—i.e., there is sample-to-sample variability—and any sample would also not have the same mean as that of the population from which the sample was drawn. The difference between the sample characteristic and that of the population is the sampling error. In other words, the sampling error is the difference in size between the sample estimate and the population parameter. The SD is a *descriptive statistic* and a *point estimate* that quantifies the variation in measurements for a *variable* in a sample but cannot provide a measure of the sampling error. Yet, the sampling error can be quantified with the SE. The SE describes the precision of the sample statistic—in our case, the mean—as an estimate of the population mean. The SD reflects the variability of individual data points, while the SE is the variability of, in our example, the sample means. As the population parameter is unknown, the sampling error cannot be measured accurately, but the SE can estimate the uncertainty—that is, make an inference—of the sampling error. But there are other important differences between SD and SEM.

First, scores used to calculate SD represent individual measurements of one sample (e.g., mean height), while scores used to calculate SEM represent data from several studies (e.g., mean heights from several studies). Second, SD is a descriptive statistic that will inform us about the variability in a sample that will apply only to members of the population from which the data were collected, while the SE is an inferential statistic that will generalize how far a sample mean is from the actual population mean. Third, when we calculate an SD, we use actual measured scores that show the variation of the sample, but SEM is a calculated estimate of variation based on what we would have found if we had repeated the same study multiple times. Fourth, SD can approximate how far a score in a sample is from the population mean, but as we do not know the population mean, this information is very limited. However, the SEM can help and quantify the precision—with a confidence interval—by which we can infer what the actual population mean might be. For example, we can randomly draw a sample of 100 men from the population of men in NYC and then calculate their mean height. An SD will describe the variability (dispersion) of our sample but is not an inferential statistic. The SEM, on the other hand, will derive the difference of means from this and similarly drawn samples (e.g., if 50 samples of the same size had randomly been drawn for the population of men in New York City) and estimate the difference between the mean heights of such samples and the actual mean height of all men in the city. As SEM estimates the differences between sample means, SEM informs us how confident we should be when representing the average of a whole population based on data generated by sample means. Fifth, SEM is always smaller than SD, as SEM is the quotient of SD and the square root of the sample size (Appendix 1, Formula 4.1).

- Some study authors report their results like this: "112.55 ± 4.3," where 112.55 is the mean and 4.3 is some measure of variability. It will be impossible to know if 4.3 is the SD or SEM. It is best practice to report whether the number that comes after the plus-minus symbol refers to the SD or SEM or some other measure of variability.
- Standard error is used in calculations for confidence intervals (Appendix 1, Formula 4.2).
- Similar to SD, which can be depicted in a *normal distribution* (Chapter 3), SEM can be depicted in a similar distribution, called the *sampling distribution of the mean*. While the normal distribution displays the frequency of each score in a sample (the y-axis), a mean of all scores observed in a sample (the middle of the x-axis), and SDs surrounding the mean (the x-axis), the sample distribution of the mean has similar characteristics. In this distribution, the frequency of each hypothetical sample mean is analogous to the frequency of each score in a sample in a normal distribution (the y-axis); a mean of all sample means is analogous to the mean of all scores observed in a normal distribution (the middle of the x-axis); and the SEM is analogous to the SD in a normal distribution (the x-axis). Importantly, in a normal standard distribution the mean is 0 and is surrounded by the standard deviations, but in a sampling distribution of the mean, the mean is equal to the population mean. SEM can be used in a sampling distribution of the mean in similar manners as SD is used in a normal distribution where 68.27% of sample means are clustered 1 SEM around the mean of the distribution and 95% of sample means are clustered 1.96 SEM around the mean of the distribution (Chapter 3). We can assume that the sampling distribution of continuous variables, such as sample means, follows a *normal distribution* (Chapter 3) regardless of the shape (e.g., skewed distribution) of the underlying population distribution. This assumption holds true when, in general, the sample size is above 30. This phenomenon is known as the *central limit theorem*. Larger sample sizes produce smaller SEMs and in turn more precise estimates of *effects* (i.e., the spread of mean values along the x-axis gets narrower as sample size increases) (Figure 4.2).

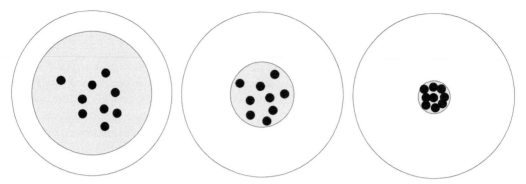

Figure 4.2 Relationship between precision and confidence interval. The smaller the area to "capture" all shots that have been made, the more precise shooting. The smaller the area, i.e., the more narrow the confidence interval generated from the observed data, the more precise is the result. Choosing a confidence interval with a larger confidence coefficient, e.g., choosing a 99% instead of a 95% confidence interval, does not increase precision, it only increases or, if choosing a confidence interval with a with a smaller confidence coefficient, decreases your confidence that you will "capture" all shots that will be made.

- Apart from SEM and SE of a sample proportion, there are two other statistical concepts using the words "standard error"—the *standard error of the estimate* and the *standard error of measurement*.

    The **standard error of the estimate** is related to regression analysis (Chapter 11) and reflects the variability around the estimated regression line and the accuracy of the regression model. Similar to SEM, the standard error of the estimate can be used to construct a *confidence interval* for the *regression coefficient*.

    The **standard error of measurement** indicates the variability of the measurement error of a test and is often reported in standardized testing. The standard error of measurement can also be used to create a confidence interval for the actual score of an element or an individual.

An application of standard error to a hair loss problem

Ronald is a very vain man who is concerned with his emerging hair loss, which he notices when brushing his hair—several strands of hair are stuck to the brush each time. He decides to count the number of hairs on his brush every day for a week. Seeing that he does lose hair every day, he decides to seek a remedy.

To prevent his hair loss, he starts every morning with eating Håravfall Yogurt with some secret ingredients that he had read about on the internet. Unfortunately, this yogurt is very expensive. Despite its shockingly high price, Ronald decides to eat one serving every morning for 20 weeks and measure whether the yogurt has any effect by counting the number of hairs on his brush every day. He forwards all the data he collects to his older brother, Aylmer, who happens to be a statistical maven.

Aylmer looks at the data and notices daily variability in the samples—ranging from 100 to 500 strands of hair every day. With the data Ronald provided, Aylmer calculated a range of strands of hair lost every week, which he presented to Ronald. He also informed Ronald that he is 95% certain that the range of number of hair strands lost in each of the 20 weeks contains the actual ("true") average hair loss. The problem is, he doesn't know which week's range didn't contain the actual average hair loss.

Ronald was not happy with these results because he wanted to know if the high expense he incurred when buying Håravfall Yogurt could be accommodated within his very strict weekly budget. Knowing that there would be some variability in the average hair loss if Ronald tried the yogurt for many additional 20-week intervals, which Ronald really couldn't justify without surrendering some other important budget item, Aylmer made another calculation. Aylmer could now inform Ronald that based on his new calculation, he is 95% confident that Ronald will lose between 102 to 298 strands of hair every week and he is 50% confidence that Ronald will lose between only 66 to as many as 234 strands of hair every week. As Aylmer only had one sample from which to work with, his standard error will be the same for any confidence interval he constructs based on this single sample. However, even when using the same standard error the confidence level will affect the confidence interval (Chapter 6). Based on this disappointing result, Ronald decided to choose another hair loss remedy.

Selected readings

Greenland S, Senn SJ, Rothman KJ, et al. Statistical tests, *P* values, confidence intervals, and power: a guide to misinterpretations. *Eur J Epidemiol.* 2006;31(4):337–350.

Macaskill P. Standard deviation and standard error: interpretation, usage and reporting. *Med J Aust.* 2018;208(2):63–64.

McManus IC. Misinterpretation of the standard error of measurement in medical education: a primer on the problems, pitfalls and peculiarities of the three different standard errors of measurements. *Med Teach.* 2012;34(7):569–576.

Sedgwick P. Standard deviation or standard error on the mean. *BMJ.* 2015;350:h831.

5

Understanding and interpreting hypothesis testing and p-values

Many studies in medicine, dentistry, and other areas in the biomedical disciplines focus on *outcomes* relevant to clinical practice. These studies may compare how well certain medications work, examine disease *risk* reduction, measure side effects associated with specific interventions, and much more. However, it is essential to differentiate between *statistically significant* results and *clinically significant* results (Chapter 20). In this chapter the concepts underlying statistical significance are addressed.

Descriptive and inferential statistics

To understand and benefit from study results, the resultant data must be tabulated, analyzed, and presented. The most common approach to the synthesis of data in biomedical research is using *descriptive statistics* and *inferential statistics*. Descriptive statistics are used to report actual findings from a *sample* without making any inference about how they can be generalized to other groups. For example, we can examine the caries rate among teenagers in a specific high school and then report the rate without analyzing how this rate might mirror that in another group of teenagers.

Inferential statistics are rooted in the ability to infer (derive, surmise) from a sample what might be observed in another group or in an entire *population*. For example, a study of bone loss after using a particular implant in a group of individuals could be used to infer the expected mean bone loss in other groups of individuals who have received the same implant. Inferential statistics can be subdivided into two complementary parts: estimation and hypothesis testing. Estimation refers to estimating (assessing) *population parameters* from *sample statistics*, with *point estimates* and *interval estimates* like *confidence intervals* (Chapter 6), while *statistical hypothesis testing* refers to examining whether data obtained in a study—a sample statistic—support a hypothesis that there exists a difference between the sample statistic and some population parameter or whether sample statistics are different from each other.

The progression of scientific knowledge is based on theories or hypotheses that are tested; statistical hypothesis testing is the dominant practice in biomedical research.

Descriptive statistics involve only a description of data from a drawn sample; descriptive statistics are not associated with any uncertainty. In contrast, inferential statistics are associated with uncertainties as a drawn sample is used to estimate or surmise information about the study population. Estimates from inferential statistics are based on many different assumptions about the sample and the sampling, such as the following: Were individuals in the sample appropriately selected and assigned? Does the sample contain the specific characteristic of interest? Was the statistical analysis used to summarize the sample statistic appropriate? As we make numerous assumptions, many uncertainties associated with inferential statistics need to be addressed.

Sampling error

A sample mean (a sample statistic) is most likely different from the mean for the population (the population parameter) from which the sample was drawn. The difference between the sample statistic and the parameter is known as *sampling error* (Chapter 1). Minimizing sampling error is a vital aspect of inferential statistics. Strategies to minimize sampling error include prestudy considerations such as sample size (Chapter 7) and employing methods to minimize differences between the sample characteristics and the population characteristics, such as the selection of study participants in a randomized manner (Chapter 1). After sample data have been collected, statistical analyses are used to estimate how confident we are that our sample reflects the population (Chapter 6). However, as the "true" population parameter is usually unknown, we never know the actual sampling error. The best we can do is estimate the sampling error and factor it into the presentation of study results. As sampling error is always expected, statistical hypothesis testing assesses the sample statistics and estimates the sampling error to determine if the observed data support a specific hypothesis.

Consider this example of sampling error when a population parameter is known:

> We know that when flipping a fair coin we have a 50% chance, or *probability*, of getting a head and a 50% chance of getting a tail (population parameter = 0.5). Thus, if we flip a fair coin 40 times, we should expect to get 20 heads and 20 tails. However, when I did the experiment with a fair coin, I got 28 heads and 12 tails. My sample statistic for the chance of obtaining a head was $0.7 \left(\frac{28}{40} = 0.7 \right)$. The difference between my sample statistic (0.7) and the population parameter (0.5) was 0.2. This is the sampling error.

Hypothesis testing or null hypothesis significance testing

There are five steps integral to hypothesis testing—two prestudy steps and three additional poststudy steps:

- Prestudy steps:
  1) State the null hypothesis and the alternative hypotheses
  2) Select a level of significance
- Poststudy steps:
  1) Perform the study, collect and summarize the sample data
  2) Analyze the observed (obtained) data
  3) Make a decision to reject or not reject the null hypothesis

Null and alternative hypotheses

The basic tenet of hypothesis testing is to estimate if a difference exists between the *distribution* of values in a sample and the distribution in the population; or, when comparing two samples, if the distributions in the two samples differ. If a difference exists between a sample and a population, or between two different samples, is the observed difference sufficient to claim that the sample came from a particular population or that the two samples came for the same population?

The null hypothesis is the assumption that no difference exists between our sample and the population. A null hypothesis is usually denoted as H_0, and we can write a no-difference as $H_0 : \mu = \bar{x}$, where μ represents the population mean and $\bar{x}$ (x-bar) represents the sample mean. An alternative hypothesis (H_A or H_1) is an alternative to the null hypothesis. When assessing the probability of observing a result, there are two options: (1) the combined probability that the observed value or a more extreme value could occur in both directions from zero, that is, higher or lower; (2) the probability that the observed value or a more extreme value occurs either as only higher or only lower than zero. The former is referred to as a two-tailed hypothesis, the latter as a one-tailed hypothesis (Figures 5.1a and 5.1b). Thus, the null hypothesis in a two-tailed hypothesis study is that there is no difference, and the null hypothesis in a one-tailed hypothesis study is that the observed result is not larger than no difference or, alternatively, not smaller than no difference.

Consider this example:

> If we calculated the mean height of a group of 25-year-old men randomly selected from all men in the United States, can we claim that our sample mean is not different from the mean height of men playing in the National Basketball Association (NBA)? Assume that study participants were randomly selected and the study was appropriately conducted.

To proceed according to the five steps delineated above, in step 1 we wanted to know if the mean height of our sample ($\bar{x}$) differed from that of NBA players (μ). The null hypothesis is thus that

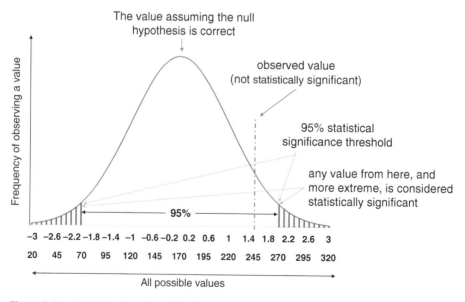

Figure 5.1a Two-tailed hypothesis testing.

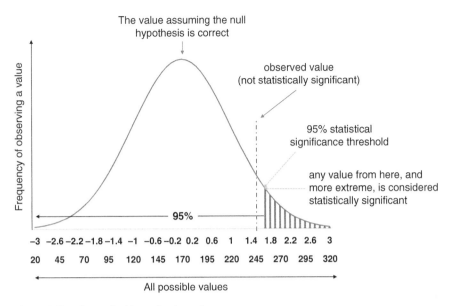

Figure 5.1b   One-tailed hypothesis testing.

there is no difference in the mean height among the men in our sample compared with that of NBA players ($\bar{x} = \mu$). We can choose three different alternative hypotheses (H_A): (1) that there is a difference and the mean height in our group was shorter or was taller than that of NBA players—a two-tailed hypothesis $\left(H_A : \bar{x} \neq \mu\right)$. However, we could also have other alternative hypotheses, such as (2) our group of men were on average taller than NBA players $\left(H_A : \bar{x} > \mu\right)$ or (3) our group of men were on average shorter than NBA players $\left(H_A : \bar{x} < \mu\right)$, two different one-tailed hypotheses.

For step 2, before conducting the study, we decided that if our observed data or even more extreme data (even shorter mean height) were less than 5% of what would have been found among NBA players, we would reject our null hypothesis. The 5% is our predetermined significance level, which is a number defined by the researcher indicating the cutoff for an observed result to be statistically significant (Figures 5.1a, 5.1b). In step 3, we measured the height of each male in our sample and found the mean to be 71 inches. In step 4, we compared our observed data with those regarding the average height of male NBA players (78 inches) and estimated that there was a 0.99% or less chance that our observed mean height (71 inches), or an even lower mean height, is the mean height of men playing in the NBA (Figure 5.2). For step 5, we concluded that our sample of men was not drawn from a group of NBA players and rejected the null hypothesis that the mean height of men in our sample is the same as the mean height of men playing in the NBA.

Significance

Based on our predetermined significance level and our observed data, the null hypothesis is either rejected or not. If the observed data support rejecting the null hypothesis, we claim a statistically significant finding; if not, our finding will be reported as statistically not significant. Importantly, statistical significance is a dichotomized concept—it exists or doesn't. What we are assessing when conducting hypothesis testing is the probability of being able to reject or not reject a stated null hypothesis.

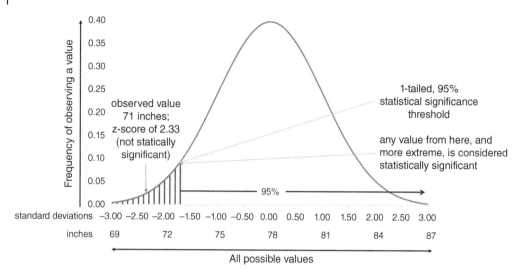

Figure 5.2 Average height of male NBA players is 78 inches with a standard deviation of 3 inches. Our sample of males had an average height of 71 inches, which equals a z-score of 2.33 (Appendix 1, Formula 3.1a). A z-score of 2.33 equals 0.9901 (Appendix 2). Thus, only 1-0.9901=0.0099 or 0.99 % of male NBA basketball players are estimated to be 71 inches or more extreme (even less than 71 inches).

P-value

Consider the following example:

> In a hypothetical study a new local anesthetic is evaluated to determine if it performs better than a traditional local anesthetic in achieving numbness. The researchers hypothesize that the new local anesthetic will be better than the traditional one at achieving numbness (one-tailed hypothesis). The study is performed according to acceptable research methods. Two groups of volunteers are randomly recruited and randomly assigned, with 95 individuals in each group—one receiving the new anesthetic, the other receiving the traditional anesthetic. In the group that receives the traditional local anesthetic, 62 report numbness (65.3%), while in the group that receives the new local anesthetic 48 report numbness (50.5%). Based on these observed outcomes, it is concluded that the traditional anesthetic is better than the new anesthetic with a one-tailed p-value of 0.02 (Appendix 1, Equation 5.1, Equation 5.2). This p-value was calculated based on the observed study data using specific statistical tests. A critical level of significance—the cutoff between a statistically significant finding and a statistically nonsignificant finding—was predetermined to be <0.05 (<5%). Because 0.02 is less than 0.05, the traditional local anesthetic was determined to be statistically significantly better than the new local anesthetic.

The most misinterpreted and misunderstood index in the biomedical literature is the p-value. Essentially, a p-value is used in hypothesis testing to assess the probability that an observation is either important or unimportant. But there are fundamental caveats to this statement that need to be clarified and understood.

What does this really mean?

One problem with the p-value is its counterintuitive nature. A hypothesis is a statement about a particular quandary that could possibly, but not always, be tested to see if it is true (should not be rejected) or false (should be rejected). Hypothesis testing involves formulating two hypotheses—the alternative (research) hypothesis and the null hypothesis. The alternative hypothesis is based on what we want to study—in this case, whether the new local anesthetic is better, as measured by reported numbness, than the traditional local anesthetic. The null hypothesis, or more accurately the "null hypothesis of no difference," is the hypothesis that there is no (null) difference between the effects of the two studied local anesthetics. The p-value does not "test" the alternative hypothesis but rather provides a measure that allows us to either fail to reject or reject the null hypothesis. Informally, the p-value is the probability of obtaining the observed result (the summary of the sample data), *assuming* that the null hypothesis is true. Importantly, a p-value cannot confirm a hypothesis; it can only assess the significance by comparing the observed data to a null hypothesis from a statistical perspective and cannot make claims of clinical significance. By clinical significance, we mean a magnitude of effect that is relevant for patients and clinicians to the point of considering a change in practice (Chapter 20).

The observed differences in the example above may be due to the traditional anesthetic actually being better than the new anesthetic in achieving numbness, or the observed difference may be due to other reasons, such as how the statistical model was built—how the data were collected and analyzed, how the results of the study were presented, and other assumptions, many of which include assumptions of chance due to data variability. Thus, although we can "reject" the null hypothesis, we cannot "accept" the alternative hypothesis, as there theoretically could be numerous different alternative hypotheses to the one and only null hypothesis.

Let's assume that the null hypothesis (that there is no difference between the effects of the two studied local anesthetics) is true; then the smaller the p-value, the greater the statistical incompatibility of the observed outcomes (a difference between the effects of the two anesthetics) with the null hypothesis—in other words, the less likely it is that reasons *other than* the actual effect generated the observed difference. Only if all our assumptions surrounding the statistical model used in the study are correct can we claim that a smaller p-value corresponds to stronger evidence. However, it is very unlikely that all our assumptions are correct, and thus assigning a modifier, such as stronger or weaker evidence, is not recommended.

The result of a study is designated as "statistically significant" when the calculated p-value is below a predetermined cutoff or level of significance, which suggests that we can reject the null hypothesis as there is scant evidence (a p-value below the predetermined cutoff) to not reject it. If the calculated p-value is above the predetermined critical cutoff value, we call the research finding "statistically not significant" and we do not reject the null hypothesis. There is evidence (a p-value above the predetermined threshold) to not reject the null hypothesis. In essence, statistical significance reflects the improbability of our findings. Importantly, as mentioned above, statistical significance doesn't equate to clinical or even scientific significance.

In the example above, assuming the null hypothesis is true (that there is no difference between the effects of the two studied local anesthetics), a p-value of 0.02 means that there is only a 2% chance that the observed difference between the two anesthetics ($65.3\% - 50.5\% = 14.8$ percentage points) could have been observed even if the traditional anesthetic was *not better* than the new local anesthetic. In other words, there is a 2% chance that reasons other than the actual different effect between the two types of anesthetics can explain the observed data. Note that a p-value of <0.05 doesn't mean that the traditional anesthetic is truly better than the new anesthetic; it means only that we have enough evidence to reject the null hypothesis, that is, that the new anesthetic is no different from the traditional anesthetic.

A few additional notes

- Why do we use the null hypothesis? The scientific process is based on the notion that a scientific hypothesis is believed to be correct until it can be disproved. Many different types of studies can be performed to confirm a hypothesis, but a single study is sufficient to reject one. Take the alternative hypothesis that only white swans exist. The null hypothesis is that black swans exist. Let's assume we live in a region with 1,000 white swans and only one black swan. Every time we try to assess the swan population, by selecting a sample from the entire population, we are likely to find that there are only white swans, but only one single study showing evidence of the existence of a black swan would be enough to reject the hypothesis that black swans don't exist.

- Why use 0.05 for the level of significance? There is really no scientific rationale for why 0.05 or 5% is commonly used in the biomedical literature. In fact other levels of significance, such as 1%, are sometimes used. In genome-wide association studies, a significance level as small as $<10^{-8}$ is a common threshold to establish statistical significance.

- A common mistake is to add a modifier to the p-value. If the predetermined level of a significance of <0.05 is used to determine the statistical significance of a study outcome, the only statement that can be made, after having calculated a p-value, is that the observed outcome is statistically significant or not significant. The outcome cannot be "almost" significant (e.g., a p-value of 0.048), "marginally" significant (e.g., a p-value of 0.052), or highly significant (e.g., a p-value < 0.0001). Furthermore, a p-value should never be reported as $p = 0.00$, as there is always, even if infinitesimally small, some possibility of observing our data.

- It is incorrect to claim that a p-value of 0.04 has only a 4% chance of the null hypothesis being true. As the p-value is calculated based on a statistical model that *assumes that the null hypothesis is true*, the p-value cannot at the same time represent the probability that the null hypothesis is false, that is, being rejected.

- In our hypothetical case described above, there is a probability of 2% that the observed difference of 14.8 percentage points, or greater, would have been observed *if* all underlying assumptions, including the null hypothesis, were correct. As statistical models already include an assessment of chance, we cannot claim that the p-value is the probability that chance, or chance alone, produced the observed association.

- A statistically nonsignificant finding, such as $p = 0.06$ when the critical cutoff value for significance is <0.05, does not mean there is no difference between the groups being studied. A nonsignificant finding can inform us only that the null effect (no difference) is statistically consistent with the observed summary data. When researchers fail to reject the null hypothesis, basically we will continue perceive the world through the premise of the null hypothesis.

- The predetermined cutoff value used to determine the statistical threshold for significance is usually represented with the Greek letter α (*alpha*).

- The effect is the difference between the true population parameter and the null hypothesis value.

- Lastly, we can get different p-values but the same measure of effect. Consider the following hypothetical example. Two studies were performed to compare diastolic blood pressure (DBP), each with two groups of participants (G_1 and G_2). In study 1, with 30 participants, the mean DBP values in the two groups were 105.0 mm Hg and 108.5 mm Hg, respectively, and the p-value for the mean difference in DBP between the groups was 0.417 (Appendix 1, Equation 5.3). In study 2, also with 30 participants, the mean DBP values in the two groups were also 105.0 mm Hg and 108.5 mm Hg, respectively, but the p-value for the mean difference in DBP between the groups was 0.019 (Appendix 1, Equation 5.4). The only difference between the studies was their respective standard deviations (Chapter 3). Thus, looking only at different p-values cannot tell us anything about a difference in the size of an effect; in this case the size of the effect was the same—a mean difference of –3.5 mm Hg.

- In summary, a p-value is of little value when assessing a clinically important outcome, and many scientific journals request that researchers avoid using a p-value as a metric for the importance of their clinical research findings.

An application of null and alternative hypotheses to soccer referees' calls

In many athletic venues today, there is an option to review a referee's call of a foul or an infraction. For example, in soccer, a call was made that a player was offside. The call was challenged, so the referee reviewed all available evidence to determine if there was enough evidence to reverse her call. She reviewed the play with the help of slow-motion recordings that she could play forward and backward, and she also viewed recordings of the incident from different angles. After having viewed all available evidence, the referee had two choices—either reject and reverse her initial call or not reject the initial call. As she initially called the offside, this is her alternative hypothesis, while reversing (rejecting) the initial call is the null hypothesis. If we assume that the referee is schooled in statistics, she will choose a predetermined threshold, for example 5%, which she uses to determine if there is enough evidence to reverse (reject) her initial call. In other words, if she determines based on the observed evidence that there are less than 5% evidentiary reasons to reverse her initial call, she will reject this hypothesis and her initial call will not be reversed.

If she is 75% certain that she should reverse her call, she will reverse her call and not reject her null hypothesis. If she is 10% certain that she should reverse her call, she will reverse her call and not reject her null hypothesis. But if she is only 4% percent certain, based on the observed data, that her initial call should be reversed, she concludes that there is not enough evidence to reverse her initial call and rejects her null hypothesis (she rejects reversing her initial call).

Instead of looking at the evidence to substantiate her initial call, she looked at how certain she would be to reverse her initial call. If she wasn't very certain, only 4% certainty that there was enough evidence to reverse her call, she doesn't reverse her call. She used a cutoff for this determination of <5%. This is the equivalence of having a p-value below a predetermined cutoff value, which would result in a decision to reject the null hypothesis. Please note, she will never state if her initial call was correct, only if there was enough or not enough evidence to reverse or not reverse her initial call.

Selected readings

Best AM, Greenberg BL, Glick M. From tea tasting to *t* test: a *p* value ain't what you think it is. *J Am Dent Assoc.* 2016;147(7):527–529.

Greenland S, Senn SJ, Rothman KJ, et al. Statistical tests, P values, confidence intervals, and power: a guide to misinterpretations. *Eur J Epidemiol.* 2016;31:337–350.

Sedgwick P. What is significance? *BMJ.* 2015;350:h3475.

6

Understanding and interpreting a confidence interval

Statistical models are used in biomedical research to draw conclusions from *sample* data in order to generalize the observed results to other individuals or *populations*. For example, we want to know the average DMFT (diseased, missing, filled teeth) among teenagers in New York City (NYC). One method to acquire these data would be to examine every teenager who resides there. Obviously, such an endeavor is unrealistic, so instead we can select a representative sample of teenagers and use the data from these teenagers to infer what the data would look like if we had examined every teenager in the city. Unfortunately, such an inference can never be made with absolute certainty, so we need to present our data together with an estimate of our certainty of, or our confidence in, our summary of results. One way of accomplishing this is to use a *confidence interval* (CI). Informally, a CI is an estimation of how well sample data can be generalized, presented with a lower and an upper limit, with a specified degree of confidence.

Consider the following example:

> To determine the DMFT score among a population of teenagers in NYC, we recruit and examine a random sample of 83 teenagers, selected and examined according to acceptable research methods and analyzed with the appropriate statistical model. The *mean* (average) DMFT score is 4.25 DMFT, with a *standard deviation* of 1.64 (Chapter 3). The calculated 95% CI surrounding this mean is the mean minus 0.35 (4.25 − 0.35 = 3.90) and the mean plus 0.35 (4.25 + 0.35 = 4.60), which can be written as "mean (95% confidence interval [CI]); 4.25 DMFT (95% CI; 3.90 DMFT to 4.60 DMFT)" (Appendix 1, Equation 6.1a, Figure 6.1).

To calculate a CI for a mean, we need to determine our level of confidence (95%, 90%, or any other level we feel is appropriate), know the standard deviation of our sample, and know the number of participants (Appendix 1, Formula 6.1a-l). With this information we can estimate the *margin of error* (ME) (Appendix 1, Formula 6.1b-f), which represents the amount we think the true population value is from our point estimate (a point estimate is a single value, not a range of values, representing the population—in our case all teenagers in NYC) given our chosen level of confidence. In our example, the ME is ±0.35 (Appendix 1, Equation 6.1b). We constructed our CI around the point estimate by adding and subtracting the ME from the point estimate. The width of a CI is a measure of *precision*—or the degree of certainty we have in the sample statistic we estimated. The smaller the width or range of the estimated interval, the more precise the estimate, while the larger the width or range, the less precise the estimate (Figure 4.2). The precision is determined by the standard error (Chapter 4).

Statistics for Dental Clinicians, First Edition. Michael Glick, Alonso Carrasco-Labra, and Olivia Urquhart.
© 2024 John Wiley & Sons, Inc. Published 2024 by John Wiley & Sons, Inc.

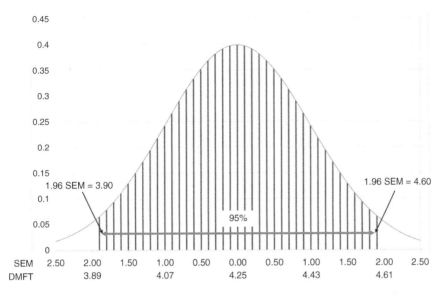

Figure 6.1   95% confidence interval depicted within a normal distribution. SEM - standard error of the mean, DMFT - diseased, missing, filled teeth, n - sample size; mean = 4.25 DMFT, standard deviation = 1.64, n = 83; mean (95% confidence interval [CI]); 4.25 DMFT (3.90 DMFT to 4.60 DMFT) (Appendix 1, Equation 6.1a).

Understanding the confidence interval

Unlike a p-value, which can inform us only if we can or cannot reject a null hypothesis (Chapter 5), a CI provides information about both direction (i.e., improvement or deterioration, increase or decline) and magnitude of the effect (how large the DMFT score or how much a treatment improved a disease).

Importantly, the *confidence coefficient*, a measure of a CI accuracy, (e.g., 95%) is not the probability of our CI containing the population parameter. In our example, there is not a 95% chance (probability) that the population mean is between 3.90 and 4.60. Instead, a 95% CI should be interpreted as a 95% probability that our particular estimated CI—which is the only one we have but is one among all theoretical 95% CIs that could have been estimated if exactly the same sampling method was used to draw samples from the same population—is one that contains the population parameter. In other words, if 100 samples were drawn—with the same method and from the same population—and 100 CIs were constructed around these sample means, 95% of the CIs would contain the true population parameter and 5% of the CIs would not (Figure 6.2). The problem is, we don't know if our specific calculated 95% CI (3.90–4.60) is one of the 95% CIs that contain the population mean DMFT or one of the 5% CIs that do not. In summary, according to what we found among this random sample of 83 teenagers, we can state that if we performed the exact same study 99 additional times, 95% of the CIs would contain the actual mean DMFT score of all teenagers in NYC (the actual average DMFT score refers to the mean DMFT score we would have observed if we had examined every teenager in the city).

How to interpret a confidence interval

Unlike a p-value, a CI can be used to assess clinical significance (Chapter 20) (Table 6.1). Let's assume that we instituted a caries-prevention program. In order to ascertain if the program was clinically successful, we performed a study. We decided that the program was successful if the

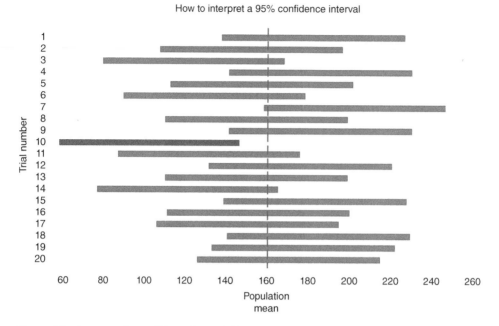

Figure 6.2 Accuracy of a confidence interval. If we measured the weight of the same number of people, in the same manner, from the same population 20 times, and constructed a 95% confidence interval (CI) around every sample mean, 19 (95%) of the CIs would contain the actual population mean, in this example 160 lbs, and 1 (5%) would not contain the population mean. However, a research trial usually only measures a single sample, with a single corresponding CI, and we do not know if this particular CI contains the population mean. Yet, we can state that we are 95% confident that our particular CI contains the population mean.

Table 6.1 Assessing statistical significance using confidence intervals and p-values.

Parameter	Null value	Assessing significance using the CI	Assessing significance using the corresponding p-value
Difference: mean difference, standardized mean difference, risk difference, rate difference	0	Confidence interval contains 0 = nonsignificant	$P \geq 0.05$
		Confidence interval does not contain 0 = significant	$P < 0.05$
Ratio: relative risk, odds ratio, risk ratio	1	Confidence interval contains 1 = nonsignificant	$P \geq 0.05$
		Confidence interval does not contain 1 = significant	$P < 0.05$

© 2019 American Dental Association. Used with permission. All rights reserved.
Glick M, Greenberg BL. Primer to biostatistics for busy clinicians. In: Carrasco-Labra A, Brignardello-Petersen A, Glick M, Azarpazooh A, Guyatt G, eds. *How to Use Evidence-Based Dental Practice to Improve Your Clinical Decision-Making.* American Dental Association Publishing; 2020:185–208.

DMFT is below 4.00. This threshold of clinical significance was determined prior to performing the study and took into consideration a number of factors, but mostly focusing on the following: what is the minimum benefit in DMFT reduction that a population or a patient can perceive from the caries-prevention program to justify the costs, health care system burden, and patient adverse events? Instead of 83 participants as in the last example, we instead sample 159 participants (the

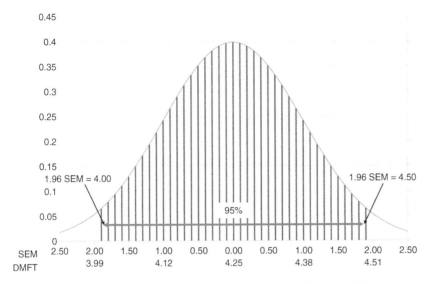

Figure 6.3 95% confidence interval depicted within a normal distribution. SEM - standard error of the mean, DMFT - diseased, missing, filled teeth, n - sample size; mean = 4.25 DMFT, standard deviation = 1.64, n = 159; mean (95% confidence interval [CI]); 4.25 DMFT (4.00 DMFT to 4.50 DMFT) (Appendix 1, Equation 6.2).

number calculated based on a statistical model to assess an appropriate sample size (Chapter 7). The mean DMFT after the implementation of the caries-prevention program was 4.25 DMFT, 95% CI (4.00 DMFT to 4.50 DMFT) (Appendix 1, Equation 6.2, Figure 6.3). As the lower limit of the CI did not go below the predetermined clinically relevant level of DMFT of 4.00, the program was deemed unsuccessful. It is very important to consider both the lower and upper limits of CIs when assessing clinical or practical importance of an *outcome* variable (Chapter 20).

A few additional notes

- In our example, we selected a CI of 95%, but we could also have selected 90%, which would have given us less confidence, or 99%, which would have increased our confidence, or any other CI value. A 90% CI, surrounding the same mean and with the same standard deviation in a sample of 80 participants, would have given us an interval of 3.95 to 4.55 (Appendix 1, Equation 6.3, Table 6.2a), while a 99% CI would have given us an interval of 3.78 to 4.72 (Appendix 1, Equation 6.4, Table 6.2a).
- When we look for more confidence, we sacrifice precision as we get a wider interval (larger ME) with a higher (99% CI, n = 80, ME = 0.94) (Appendix 1, Equation 6.4, Table 6.2a) compared with a lower (95% CI, n = 80, ME = 0.36) level of confidence even when we keep the same sample (Table 6.2a).
- Another choice we made was to select a sample of 80 teenagers, but we could also have decided to select 20, 320, or any other number of teenagers. The number of participants selected for a study is largely based on feasibility factors (e.g., cost, time, availability of examiners). How would the CI change if we selected a smaller or a larger sample but kept the same confidence coefficient (95%)?

    Let's assume that a sample of 20 teenagers would have produced the same mean (4.25) and standard deviation (1.64) as when we selected a sample of 80 teenagers. With only 20

Table 6.2a Confidence intervals for mean differences with different confidence coefficients and sample sizes.

	Cc	$z_{\alpha/2}$	Mean	s	n	SEM	$Z_{\alpha/2}$*SEM (ME)	CI–	CL+	Range
	90%	1.6449	4.25	1.64	20	0.37	0.60	3.65	4.85	1.21
Equation 6.3	90%	1.6449	4.25	1.64	80	0.18	0.30	3.95	4.55	0.60
	90%	1.6449	4.25	1.64	320	0.09	0.15	4.10	4.40	0.30
Equation 6.5	95%	1.9600	4.25	1.64	20	0.37	0.72	3.53	4.97	1.44
	95%	1.9600	4.25	1.64	80	0.18	0.36	3.89	4.61	0.72
Equation 6.6	95%	1.9600	4.25	1.64	320	0.09	0.18	4.07	4.43	0.36
	99%	2.5758	4.25	1.64	20	0.37	0.94	3.31	5.19	1.89
Equation 6.4	99%	2.5758	4.25	1.64	80	0.18	0.47	3.78	4.72	0.94
	99%	2.5758	4.25	1.64	320	0.09	0.24	4.01	4.49	0.47

Abbreviations: Cc—confidence coefficient; $z_{\alpha/2}$—z-score; *S*—standard deviation; SEM—standard error of the mean; ME—margin of error, CI—confidence interval.
The larger the confidence coefficient (Cc), the wider the range, the less precise is the confidence interval (CI). The ME can be decreased (more precise CI with a narrower ME) by increasing the sample size.

Table 6.2b Different confidence intervals (CIs) surrounding relative risk reduction (RRR) when keeping the RRR and the absolute risk difference (ARD) the same but changing sample sizes (Appendix 1, Equation Table 6.1b).

	a	b	c	d	Total$_{exposure}$	Total$_{control}$	RRR	ARD	RRR; CI–	RRR; CI+	Range
Study 6.1	4	16	6	14	20	20	0.33	0.10	−1.01	0.78	1.79
Study 6.2	8	32	12	28	40	40	0.33	0.10	−0.45	0.69	1.15
Study 6.3	12	48	18	42	60	60	0.33	0.10	−0.26	0.65	0.91
Study 6.4	16	64	24	56	80	80	0.33	0.10	−0.16	0.62	0.77
Study 6.5	20	80	30	70	100	100	0.33	0.10	−0.09	0.59	0.68

When the sample size increases the CI becomes more narrow even when there is no change in RRR or ARD, which is represented by the more narrow range in the last column.
For example:
Study 6.1 has an RRR of 0.33, an ARD of 0.10 and a total **sample size of 40** with RRR (95% confidence interval (CI)); 0.33 **(95% CI; −1.01 RRR to 0.78 RRR)**—range of 1.79
Study 6.3 has an RRR of 0.33, an ARD of 0.10 and a total **sample size of 120** with RRR (95% confidence interval (CI)); 0.33 **(95% CI; −0.26 RRR to 0.65 RRR)**—range of 0.91

participants in the study, the 95% CI surrounding the mean would be 3.53 to 4.97, a width of 1.44 (Appendix 1, Equation 6.5); with 320 teenagers in the sample, the 95% CI surrounding the mean would be 4.07 to 4.43, a width of 0.36 (Appendix 1, Equation 6.6). Thus, the larger the sample, the narrower the interval and the more precise the estimation. This makes sense intuitively, as the more individuals we select from a population the closer we get to the actual population value, which could be determined only by conducting a full census of the entire population of teenagers in NYC.

- Differences in sample size can also affect CI surrounding proportions, such as relative risk (Table 6.2b).

- Confidence intervals can also be used to assess statistical significance (Chapter 20). In our case, we constructed our CI around a mean as our sample *point estimate* (a point estimate is a single value, not a range of values, representing the population—in our case all teenagers in NYC). If we performed the same study among teenagers in Cleveland, we may get a different mean (a different point estimate). If our null hypothesis (Chapter 5) is that there is no difference between the two observed means and our calculated 95% CI surrounding the mean difference contains "0" (i.e., no difference), we claim our finding is not statistically significant. If the calculated 95% CI surrounding the mean difference (in our case the difference of the mean DMFT in NYC and the mean DMFT in Cleveland) does not contain "0", we claim a statistically significant finding (Table 6.1). For example, in a hypothetical study, if our calculated 95% CI surrounding the mean difference had a lower limit of –2.34 and an upper limit of 3.24 the CI contains "0" and our result is statistically not significant. However, if our calculated 95% CI surrounding the mean difference had a lower limit of 2.34 and an upper limit of 3.24 the CI doesn't contain "0" and our result is statistically significant.
- When working with proportions, such as the proportion of people in a random sample who developed periodontal disease, we can compute a CI around this point estimate. Further, if we are interested in the ratio of proportions, such as relative risk, odds ratio, or hazard ratio (Chapters 2 and 10), "no difference" means that the ratio equals 1 (the same value in both the numerator and the denominator). Thus, if our point estimate were a ratio, we would claim a lack of statistical significance if the CI contained "1" and a significant finding if the CI did not contain "1" (Table 6.1). For example, if a CI constructed around a relative risk is 0.53 to 1.47, the result is statistically not significant (the interval includes (crosses) 1), but if a CI constructed around a relative risk is 1.53 to 2.47, the result is statistically significant.
- Also, using the same statistical model (how the data were collected and analyzed, how the results of the study were presented, and other assumptions) to calculate several CIs, if two 95% CIs do not overlap, the p-value for the difference will be <0.05, that is, statistically significant. If the point estimate from one 95% CI is included in another 95% CI, the p-value of the difference will be ≥0.05, that is, statistically not significant. Importantly, although it is possible to claim a statistical significance if two confidence intervals do not overlap, it is a mistake to claim a non-statistical significance if two confidence intervals do overlap. For example, if a study was performed with two groups comparing difference of means, and the 95% CI of both groups overlapped, a claim of statistical significance cannot be made. Instead of comparing the two 95% CIs, a comparison of the actual difference of the means needs to be computed (Appendix 1, Formula 4.3, Equation 4.3). If the 95% CI of the difference of the means contains "0," no claim of statistical significance can be made; if the 95% CI of the difference of the means doesn't contain "0," a claim of statistical significance can be made (Chapter 5).

Choosing the right clothing based on different confidence intervals

We ask two people to estimate, within a given range, the average temperature in NYC in March 2020. The first person is 90% confident that the temperature ranges from 38°F to 43°F. The second person is 99% confident that the temperature ranges from 0°F to 100°F. Obviously, the second person will be more confident, more sure, that the average temperature will be contained in the wider range, making it the safer choice. However, having a wide range comes with a price. When trying to use either range to decide what to pack for the next trip to NYC in March 2021, the wider range is less precise and would force one to bring the best available winter gear (0°F) as well as a summer outfit (100°F).

Trying to estimate an average test score of fellow student

Over the past four years, on all quizzes and exams Bert has scored in the range of 10 points below to 10 points above the class average 95% of the time. On the final exam the average grade was 75. We cannot know if there is a 95% chance (probability), based on the class average, if Bert's grade was between 65 and 85 as we don't know if this was the one of the 95% of times Bert's score was in the range of 10 points below to 10 points above the class average. Maybe this was one of the 5% of times that he didn't score within 10 points below to 10 points above the class average and he scored a 92.

A 95% CI is not the same as 95% probability that the CI contains the "true" parameter.

Selected readings

Cumming G. Understanding the New Statistics: Effect Sizes, Confidence Intervals, and Meta-Analysis. Routledge; 2012.

Glick M, Greenberg BL. A march toward scientific literacy. *J Am Dent Assoc.* 2017;148(8):543–545.

Sedgwick P. Confidence intervals: predicting uncertainty. *BMJ.* 2012;344:e3147.

Sedgwick P. Confidence intervals and statistical significance: rules of thumb. *BMJ.* 2012;345:e4960.

Sedgwick P. Understanding confidence intervals. *BMJ.* 2014;349:g6051.

7

Understanding and interpreting power analysis and sample size

When researchers want to draw conclusions about a *population*, it is typically unfeasible to investigate the entire population. Instead, they select a representative *sample* from the population of interest and use data from this sample to extrapolate, or infer, what the entire population as a whole might look like. An important question that will affect how generalized research data from samples can be interpreted is this: What is the minimum sample size required to make a suitable inference, a conclusion, about the population from which the sample was drawn?

Sample size: Why is it important?

Sample size refers to the number of individuals included in a research study, whether survey-based, observational, or experimental. Depending on the type of research, the research design, and the research question, the minimum estimated sample size may differ. However, investigators must attend to basic considerations and elements common to all sample size estimations when calculating a sample size.

For example, if a sample size is too small the study may not be able to ascertain if the results reflect a "true" difference between an *intervention* and the effect of chance and such a study would therefore be a waste of resources and time and possibly needlessly expose participants to an intervention. As there is always a potential for adverse *outcomes* with any intervention trial, possible risks associated with research are justifiable only if there is a genuine chance that the study will produce useful information. A sample size that is too large is also a waste of resources and may further raise ethical concerns. If the intervention was detrimental, too many participants in the intervention group would be exposed to unnecessary harm, and if the intervention was beneficial, participants in the control group would be deprived of its benefit. Although a very large sample may provide greater precision (a smaller confidence interval; Chapter 6, Tables 6.1a and 6.1b) and statistical significance (a smaller p-value; Chapter 5) than what would have been observed with a smaller sample size, a larger sample size may be a waste of resources as a smaller sample size would have been adequate. Thus, a reader of a scientific publication must recognize how an inappropriate sample size may have affected the analysis and consequently the interpretation of the reported results. Estimating an appropriate sample size can be a challenge, but one that must be addressed and described in a research article.

Statistics for Dental Clinicians, First Edition. Michael Glick, Alonso Carrasco-Labra, and Olivia Urquhart.
© 2024 John Wiley & Sons, Inc. Published 2024 by John Wiley & Sons, Inc.

Components of a sample size calculation

There are three elements that are under the control of the investigators and need to be addressed before conducting a study to estimate an appropriate sample size—size of *effect*, *significance level* or *type I error*, and *power* or *type II error*. To better understand these concepts, assume that a *randomized controlled trial* (RCT) is conducted to ascertain if there is a difference in pain intensity after an extraction with suturing (an intervention) compared to not using any local post-extraction interventions. In this assumed "perfect" hypothetical study, all participants have the same *prognostic factors* to develop similar levels of post-extraction pain and all are given the same type and amount of pain medications to which they all respond equally.

Traditional RCTs are driven by *null hypothesis significance* testing with an *alternative hypothesis* (H_A) and a null hypothesis (H_0) (see Box 7.1 for a brief description of null hypothesis testing as well as Chapter 5 for more in-depth explanations). An alternative hypothesis proposes a relationship, usually a difference, between the values of a variable, such as pain intensity, between two or more groups (e.g., individuals with or without sutures) after an extraction, while a null hypothesis declares no relationship between the variables—that is, there is no difference in the post-extraction pain intensity experienced among individuals receiving sutures versus individuals not receiving sutures.

Size of the effect

In our hypothetical study we investigate the magnitude of the difference in the pain intensity experienced by participants in the intervention (suturing) group and by those in the non-intervention (not suturing) group. As the "true" *minimal important difference* (MID), that is,

---

Box 7.1   A brief summary of null hypothesis testing using the example of pain intensity after different post-extraction interventions described above.

For a more detailed explanation of null hypothesis testing, see Chapter 5.

Hypothesis testing (Chapter 5) is the most common type of statistical testing used in the biomedical domain when attempting to discern statistical inference from a sample and is based on the assumption that the *null hypothesis* (H_0) is true. This type of statistical testing attempts to draw a conclusion as to the veracity of the H_0 (in our example, that there is no difference in the post-extraction pain intensity after receiving or not receiving sutures) based on the observed data. In other words, H_0 is assumed to be true, and based on the observed study outcome (observed data) researchers will determine if there is enough evidence to support that there is no difference between the interventions and thus not reject H_0, or determine if there is not enough evidence to support a no difference and thus reject H_0. If, based on our preselected level of significance (e.g., using an alpha level of 5% to determine if there is enough evidence or not), H_0 is rejected, we conclude that there is a difference in post-extraction pain intensity when receiving sutures compared with not receiving sutures. Importantly, even if H_0 is rejected, H_A cannot be "accepted" as there could be other hypotheses that could explain the observed difference (Chapter 5).

Table 7.1 Sample sizes for comparing two means (Appendix 1, equations 7.1a, 7.1b, 7.2, 7.3).

Study	Size of the effect*	Power (%)	Alpha level	Sample per group	Standard deviation
1	1	80	0.05	107	2.6
2	1	80	0.01	136	2.6
3	1	90	0.05	143	2.6
4	1.5	80	0.05	48	2.6
5	1.5	80	0.01	61	2.6
6	1.5	90	0.05	64	2.6
7	2.0	80	0.05	27	2.6

* Expected difference in the mean pain intensity when receiving versus not receiving sutures after an extraction. Note how the samples sizes changes with different sizes of the effect, alpha levels (i.e., significance levels) and levels of power, all factors that are predetermined prior to performing a study. The listed sizes of effect are based on a 1 to 10 scale where, e.g. 15% would thus equal 1.5 points.

the smallest measure or value of an effect that should be both clinically meaningful and important to patients, is usually unknown, researchers need to determine what size of effect could inform practice. The clinically important effect can sometimes be gleaned from other studies, determined by experts, or guesstimated. Situations and conditions, such as the type of surgery, premedication, pain threshold, and others, can all affect the minimal clinically meaningful effect. Even though MIDs sometimes seem to be rather arbitrary, it is important to realize that if the power (see below) and *significance level* (see below) are kept constant, the smaller the size of the effect, the more difficult it is to identify a difference, and larger samples are required to find a clinical effect (if such an effect exists). Similarly, for larger effect sizes, smaller sample sizes are sufficient (Table 7.1).

Example 1. Let's make two assumptions. First, there is no difference in the post-extraction pain intensity (the null hypothesis (H_0)). Second, a difference of 10% (1 point difference in pain intensity measured using a 0 to 10 visual analog scale) is the MID; that is, a reduction of 10% is clinically meaningful and important to patients. With a prespecified significance level of 5%, a power of 80%, and an estimated pooled *standard deviation* (a combined standard deviation between the two groups) of 2.6, we should enroll 107 individuals in each group (Table 7.1, study 1; Appendix 1, Equation 7.1a). However, if we keep the significance level at 5% and the power at 80% and estimate the same pooled standard deviation as above (2.6), but we prespecify a MID of 15%, the sample size should be reduced from 107 to 48 participants in each group (Table 7.1, study 4; Appendix 1, Equation 7.1b).

Significance level and type I error

When selecting a sample from a population, we accept that there may be some variability due to chance, *confounding variables*, and other issues. Thus, before conducting a study, researchers need to determine at what level they are willing to accept a false positive or alpha (α) (rejecting the null hypothesis when the null hypothesis should not be rejected) or at what level they are willing to

Study to ascertain if there is a difference in pain intensity after an extraction if sutures are being used versus no sutures are being used.

A_S = sutures are being used; A_{NS} = no sutures are being used

Hypothesis (H_A) = A_S differs in the incidence of post-extraction pain compared with A_{NS}

Hypothesis (H_0) = There is no difference in the incidence of experiencing pain between A_S and A_{NS}

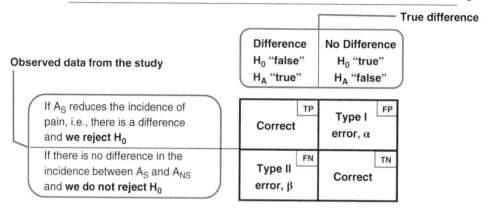

Figure 7.1 Hypothesis testing and type I and type II errors.

accept a false negative or β (not rejecting the null hypothesis when the null hypothesis should be rejected) result (Figure 7.1). In hypothesis testing, the α level is the "significance level" and 1 minus the β level $(1 - \beta)$ is the "power."

When estimating a sample size, the critical value, alpha (α), or the alpha level or significance level indicates the level for which researchers are willing to accept a false positive or reject the null hypothesis when it should not be rejected—making a type I error (Figure 7.1). In other words, if the probability of obtaining the observed data is less than the critical value of, for example, 5%, the null hypothesis is rejected, but if the probability of obtaining the observed data is greater than the predetermined critical value (α), the null hypothesis is not rejected (Chapter 5, Figures 5.1a and 5.1b).

The conventional α level is 0.05, or 5%, but α can be set at any level, such as 0.01 (1%). Another way of looking at the α level is that we accept a certain probability, say 5%, of falsely rejecting that there is no difference (the null hypothesis) (Figure 7.1). To put this probability in perspective, this level of probability is similar to the chance of getting 8 heads or more when tossing a coin 10 times. If α is set at 1%, we will reduce the chance of falsely rejecting the null hypothesis even further, where this level of probability is now similar to the chance of getting 9 or 10 heads when tossing a coin 10 times.

Falsely rejecting a null hypothesis when the null hypothesis should not be rejected (a false positive determination)—rejecting the null hypothesis when there is no difference (concluding that there is a difference when none exists)—is called making a "type I error" (Figure 7.1). Selecting an α level of 1% rather than 5% is a more cautious approach that minimizes the possibility of committing a type I error, but it will also require a larger sample size (Table 7.1, study 1 compared to study 2, and study 4 compared to study 5).

Example 2. Let's make the same assumptions as those we made in example 1. If the only element being changed is reducing the α level from 5% to 1%, the required sample size will increase from 107 to 136 individuals in each group (Table 7.1, study 1 compared with study 2; Appendix 1, equations 7.1a, 7.2).

Power and type II error

When using statistical hypothesis testing, the power of a test is the probability of correctly rejecting the null hypothesis when a difference exists. To estimate an appropriate sample size, the amount of power needs to be decided during the planning stages of the research. The reason for the use of the word "power" is that it measures the ability or the power to detect an effect if one exists. A study's power is predetermined by the researchers and is conventionally set at 80%, but it could be 85%, 90%, 95%, or any other level. If there is an 80% chance of correctly rejecting the null hypothesis (rejecting the null hypothesis when it should be rejected) (Figure 7.1), there is a 20% chance of not rejecting the null hypothesis—a false negative result. The false negative level is also known as beta (β), which is 100% minus the power (100% − power = β). Not rejecting the null hypothesis when it should be rejected is a type II error (Figure 7.1).

Example 3. Let's make the same two assumptions as those we made in example 1. If the only element being changed is the power, for example, from 80% to 90%, the required sample size will increase from 107 to 143 individuals in each group (Table 7.1; compare study 1 to study 3; Appendix 1, Equation 7.1a,7.3). The required sample size of a study increases as the power increases (Figure 7.2a).

Example 4. Let's make the first assumption as we made in example 1. If alpha and sample size are held constant, a decrease in the size of the effect will reduce the power of the study (Figure 7.2b).

H₀ - null hypothesis
Hₐ - alternative hypothesis
μ - mean
β - measure of a type II error
α - level of significance
N - sample size
SE - standard error
σ - standard deviation
1-β - power

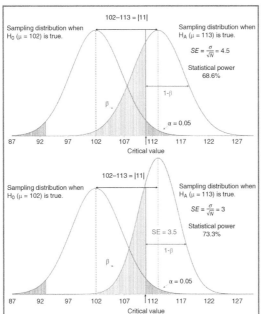

Keeping the size of the effect and the alpha constant, an increase in the sample size, which will decrease the SE, will increase the power.

Figure 7.2a Sample size and power.

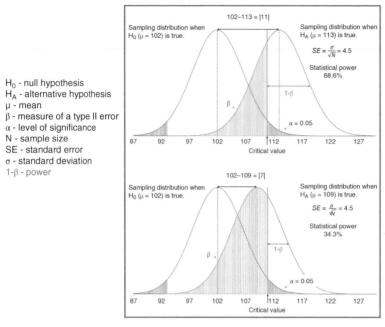

H$_0$ - null hypothesis
H$_A$ - alternative hypothesis
μ - mean
β - measure of a type II error
α - level of significance
N - sample size
SE - standard error
σ - standard deviation
1-β - power

Keeping the alpha and the sample size constant, a decrease in the size of the effect will reduce the power.

Figure 7.2b Size of an effect and power.

A few additional notes

- When standardized, the size of the effect is referred to as the *effect size* (Chapter 2).

- Depending on the study design, other factors researchers need to consider when estimating a sample size include standard deviations for *quantitative* measurements, population proportions for *categorical* measurements, *margin of error*, and attrition rate. Again, these values can be gathered from previously performed or published studies, observations from a pilot study, or expert opinion.

- To properly interpret study results, the reader must know that an appropriate sample size was used. Out of convenience or due to a lack of funding, many studies are underpowered—the sample size is too small to detect a difference between groups when one exists, a type II error. Unfortunately this is not an uncommon occurrence in the biomedical literature and should always be considered when using study results to inform clinical practice. This issue can be addressed with meta-analyses, a method in which the results of several studies are combined and analyzed in unison (Chapter 19).

- Beta and alpha levels are interdependent. Changing one level will affect the other. When an alpha level is reduced, the corresponding beta level will increase. As the beta level increases the power decreases, and the chance of detecting a difference if one exists is diminished. A similar trade-off exists when increasing the power, which will lower the beta level and increase the alpha level (Figure 7.2c). Thus, increasing the power increases the chance of getting a false positive result. Researchers must decide which is more

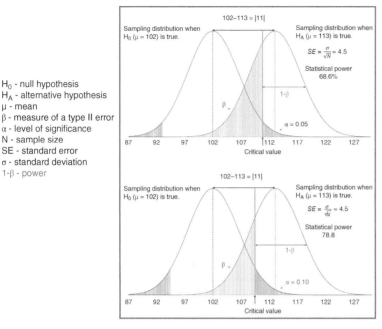

H$_0$ - null hypothesis
H$_A$ - alternative hypothesis
μ - mean
β - measure of a type II error
α - level of significance
N - sample size
SE - standard error
σ - standard deviation
1-β - power

Keeping the sample size and the size of the effect constant, an increase of the alpha will increase the power.

Figure 7.2c Alpha and power.

important—committing a type I (accepting a false positive result) or type II error (accepting a false negative result).

• The following hypothetical example illustrates the consequences of type I and type II errors.

A clinician is testing the waterlines connected to her operatory for bacterial contamination. If the bacterial load is too high, she will have to close her clinic until this issue has been rectified. Her null hypothesis is that the bacterial load is acceptable, and her alternative hypothesis is that the bacterial load is unacceptably high.

If she rejects an observed bacterial load that is acceptable she is committing type I error (rejecting the null hypothesis when it should not have been rejected; a false positive result) and will close her clinic when it is not necessary to do so.

If she does not reject an observed bacterial load that is unacceptable (too high) she is committing type II error (not rejecting the null hypothesis when it should have been rejected; a false negative result) and will not close her clinic even though it would have been necessary to do so based on the "true" bacterial load.

The more detrimental situation for her patients would be to keep her clinic open when it should have been closed (a type II error), and creating such a circumstance should preferably be avoided. Increasing her alpha level (using a higher significance level, which will make it easier reject the null hypothesis) increases her chances of making a type I error but decreases the chance of making a type II error (closing the clinic when it should have been open, rather than keeping her clinic open when it should have been closed), which is a safer situation for her patients.

- The sample size is almost always found in the denominator in formulas calculating confidence intervals, standard errors, p-values, and more. Thus, increasing the sample size will result in smaller confidence intervals and p-values, resulting in more statistically important findings. Hence, studies using sample sizes that are too large may provide a narrow and precise confidence interval, yet if a difference is found, it might not be of clinical importance.
- The β level denoting the acceptable false negative level and a type II error is not the same as a β used in other statistical calculations, such as regression analysis (Chapter 11).

Which dog to choose

You have decided that you want to get a dog. As you don't have a lot of time to walk the dog and have young children at home, you don't want to get an energetic hound who needs a lot of exercise. You stroll down to the local shelter where they have several dogs looking for a home. The person in charge, Mollis, is very knowledgeable but also has an interest in placing each dog in a home.

Here are the concerns that you must address. Most dogs are energetic. You decide that you will measure a dog's energy level according to an "energy index" ranging from 0—a very lazy lapdog that is happy laying around doing nothing all day—to 100—a dog rescued from an illegal racing ring who needs copious exercise. The dogs in the adoption center have a normal energy index distribution, with approximately two-thirds of them having an evenly distributed energy index, that is, 1 standard deviation below and 1 standard deviation above the average energy index, around the middle, which has an energy index of 50. You don't want an overly energetic dog, but you also don't want a dog that is a complete couch potato. If you decide that you are willing to have a dog with an energy index ranging from 35 to 65, you will have a larger sample to choose from than if you decide to choose a dog that has an energy index between 48 and 52.

You decide that you want a dog with an energy index of 40 and are willing to accept one with an index from 35 to 45. But you also know that you may make a mistake when choosing a dog according to your acceptable values. So you decide that you are willing to accept that there is a 5% chance of getting a dog with an index of 50 or more (type I error, α) and also willing to accept a 20% chance of getting a dog with a value of 30 or less (type II error, β).

Mollis is of course very knowledgeable but can sometimes be mistaken when it comes to assessing an energy index. You decide that Mollis can correctly determine an index 80% of the time (power), and based on this assumption you ask her to help you choose your dog. Based on all of these variables there are five dogs that fit all of your criteria. If you would change your degree of willingness to wrongly accept a more energetic dog (type I error) or wrongly agree to accept a dog with even less energy (type II error) or rely more on Mollis's advice, your sample size of eligible dogs would change accordingly.

Selected readings

Button KS, Ioannidis JPA, Mokrysz C, et al. Power failure: why small sample size undermines the reliability of neuroscience. *Nat Rev Neurosci.* 2013;14(5):365–376.

Carlin JB, Doyle LW. Statistics for clinicians. 7: Sample size. *J Paediatr Child Health.* 2002;38:300–304.

Sedgwick P. Sample size: how many participants are needed in a cohort study? *BMJ.* 2014:349:g6557.

Sedgwick P. Sample size: how many participants are needed in a trial? *BMJ.* 2013;3461:f1041.

Stokes L. Sample size calculation for a hypothesis test. *J Am Med Assoc.* 2014;312(2):180–181.

8

Understanding and interpreting a survival analysis

Clinicians and patients are interested in knowing the risk or probability of an *event* or *outcome* if they use treatment A versus treatment B or do nothing (i.e., no treatment rendered). The impact of choosing either treatment or not doing anything can be measured using a *binary or dichotomous outcome*, such as the presence or absence of a new carious lesion, dental implant failure, or aesthetic crown fracture over a specific *follow-up* time (e.g., after five years of follow-up). Binary outcomes are often reported in the research literature using a *relative risk* (RR), which provides a comparison of the *proportion* of participants experiencing the outcome or event of interest by the end of the follow-up time (e.g., determining whether an outcome occurred anytime between the start of a study and the end of follow-up) among a group of individuals receiving the intervention of interest compared to a control group (Chapter 2). When selecting an RR to present results, all events that happened during the duration of the study, regardless of when the events happened during the time of the study, are included. For example, a hypothetical study assessing dental implant failure (i.e., inability to verify osteointegration, bone loss, and mobility) after ten years of follow-up compared dental implant A to dental implant B. Results suggested that patients receiving implant A had a 10% relative reduction in the risk of experiencing implant failure compared to those receiving dental implant B (RR = 0.90). Unfortunately, this presentation of results cannot specify how may implants failed after one year, two years, three years, and so on. For example, if 20 implants were assessed in each group and in group A there was a total of 19 implant failures, but they all occurred the first year, and in group B there were also 19 implant failures, but they all occurred after 9 years, both groups have 19 implant failures after 10 years. Yet, a patient would be more interested to know how many implants failed after each year of follow-up. This information cannot be elucidated using RRs. Instead, such estimates use another measure called a *hazard ratio* (HR), often reported in *time-to-event analyses (survival analyses)*. Unlike RRs, HR measures the effect of two interventions (or *prognostic factors*) on an outcome (or event) by comparing the *risk* of an event in one group with the risk of the event in the comparison group at any time during the entire study period—the instantaneous risk or the *hazard rate* (Table 8.1). A variety of oral health outcomes, including time to relapse after orthognathic surgery, time to dental implant failure, and time to rescue analgesia, can be reported using hazard ratios.

Statistics for Dental Clinicians, First Edition. Michael Glick, Alonso Carrasco-Labra, and Olivia Urquhart.
© 2024 John Wiley & Sons, Inc. Published 2024 by John Wiley & Sons, Inc.

Table 8.1   Key concepts in survival analysis.

Key concept	Definition
Survival time	Event-free time period ending when the event of interest is observed (often an undesirable event).
Survival rate	Proportion of participants in a study not experiencing the event of interest (often an undesirable event) over everyone exposed to the treatment or prognostic factor, at a given time. It is the opposite of the hazard rate.
Survival curve	A graphical representation of the progress of a study population over time. Starting from 100% survival rate (no participants experiencing the event of interest), the curve reflects the event rate over time until all individuals have experienced the event of interest or censoring data has occurred.
Hazard rate or hazard	Also called "hazard", this is the slope of a survival curve and represents how rapidly subjects are experiencing the event of interest at any point in time. A hazard rate is also defined as the risk of having an event of interest at a particular point in time. It is the opposite of the survival rate.
Hazard ratio	A hazard ratio is a ratio of hazard rates. It is a measure of the effect of two interventions (or *prognostic factors*) on an event of interest, comparing the risk of an event in one group with the risk of the event in the comparison group at any time during the entire study period.

Kaplan–Meier or *survival curve*

A study measuring the length of a time interval until an event occurs may resemble a *continuous variable* that can be analyzed using a *t-test*, an *analysis of variance* (ANOVA) *test*, or *linear regression* (Chapter 11). To determine the length of the interval, these particular analyses require following up with participants until the outcome of interest is observed in all subjects. Any participant for whom an outcome or event of interest did not occur would be excluded from the analysis. In contrast, investigators using survival analysis consider and include all events of interest even if events are not observed in all individuals. Over a 10-year study of implant failure, some individuals could not be followed for the entire 10 years because they dropped out or disappeared after an earlier time period, say 2 years or 5 years. However, all individuals, even those with no data about implant failure, are still accounted for in the final analysis.

A *Kaplan–Meier curve* includes the duration of follow-up in units of time (e.g., months or years) on the x-axis and probability of survival, ranging from 0.0 to 1.0, on the y-axis. Figure 8.1 shows a Kaplan–Meier curve for a group of 100 individuals, each with one dental implant. The horizontal blue line is an interval and represents the *survival time* of the dental implants during that interval. At the beginning of the first interval, each of the 100 individuals (100%) have all of their implants. However, at the end of the first interval, the end of year 1, 10 implants have failed, which is represented as a sudden drop in the probability of survival or step in the curve and is, appropriately, called a *failure*. This time point is the start of the next interval.

The *cumulative probability* is defined as the product of the probability of survival from the beginning of an interval to the probability of survival at end of the interval, which is the same time point as the beginning of the next interval (Appendix 1, Formula 8.1). For example, the cumulative probability for interval 1 (between the beginning of year 1 and the end of year 1 or the beginning of year 2) is the product of the probability from the beginning of the interval, which is 1.0 (or 100% survival), and the probability of survival at the beginning of interval 2, which is 0.9 or 90% (90/100) (Appendix 1, Equation 8.1).

Interval 2 stretches from the end of year 1 to the end of year 2 (the beginning of year 3), interval 3 goes from the beginning of year 3 to the beginning of year 4.5, interval 4 goes from the beginning

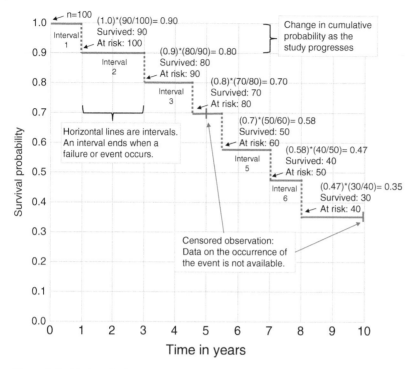

Figure 8.1 Kaplan–Meier curve showing risk estimation in every interval, cumulative probability, and the impact of censored data on a group of 100 individuals followed up for 10 years. The height of the vertical lines (red dotted lines) represents the magnitude of change in cumulative probability between two intervals. The length of the horizontal lines (blue lines) represents survival duration, which starts and ends with the occurrence of an event (failure). The calculation of the cumulative probability for every interval is indicated with small black arrows. The cumulative probability is the probability of survival from the previous interval to the probability of survival in the current interval.

of year 4.5 to the beginning of year 5.5. The small red vertical line crossing the horizontal line of interval 4 indicates that there is incomplete survival data due to the inability to observe the event of interest in some participants. In this example, 10 individuals were lost to follow-up or withdrew from the study at year 5, which in survival analysis is called *censoring*. Another type of censoring is when the event was not observed at the end of the study, in our example at the end of year 10. Thirty implants survived the entire length of the study, for which the occurrence of the event of interest (implant failure) cannot be determined. In both censoring scenarios, individuals still contributed to the analysis with the time elapsed until the censoring occurred.

Figure 8.2 represents a hypothetical study conducted between 2010 and 2020 assessing the survival of dental implants (time to implant failure) among six patients. The calendar time plot (upper graph) shows each patient on the y-axis, with a horizontal line representing their *serial time* (the period over which they were observed). The left bound of the serial time is the time they entered the study—the day a dental implant was in place. The right bound of the serial time illustrates the status of the event of interest at a particular time—for example, the time of an implant failure or of censoring. The first possibility is that the dental implant shows predetermined signs of failure, which means that the event has occurred (failure) and is represented with an X at the end of the series time (patients 1, 2, and 5). The second possibility is that although the implant was in place, the investigators were not able to observe the event of interest (censored data), represented with an O at the end

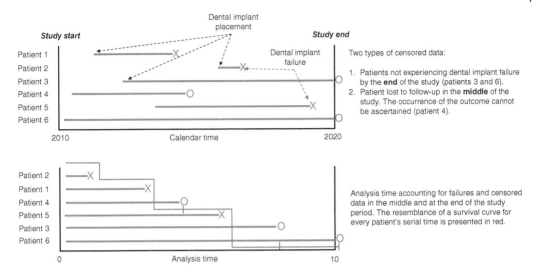

X: The outcome of interest is observed (dental implant failure); O: The outcome of interest was not observed (censored data)

Figure 8.2 Calendar and analysis time within a study assessing survival of dental implants and individual participant follow-up (serial times).

of the series time (patients 3, 4, and 6). The censored data presented in Figure 8.2 manifest in three ways: censoring due to loss to follow-up (patient 4 moved to another city), withdrawal from the study (patient 4 declined further participation), or the impossibility of observing the event of interest given that the study ended by 2020 (patients 3 and 6). After investigators complete survival data collection, they rearrange the data for analysis, which resembles the analysis time plot (lower graph). In this plot, patients' serial times are rearranged from the shortest to the longest survival regardless of when the participants entered the study and whether they have experienced a failure or their data were censored. Then, a survival curve can be plotted from left to right (curve in red).

Comparing two Kaplan–Meier (survival) curves

The survival function (the probability of surviving past a certain time or that the event of interest did not occur by the end of the study) in a group of individuals receiving an intervention can provide relevant information for practice. However, in the scientific literature it is common to see at least two Kaplan–Meier curves that are compared and plotted together.

Figure 8.3 presents the survival curves for a hypothetical study comparing two dental implants (A and B) over a 10-year period. *Median survival time* is the time elapsed for 50% of implants to have survived. In the figure, the median survival time for dental implant A is 7 years (blue dotted lines), while for implant B it is only 3.5 years (red dotted lines). This means that twice as much time will elapse before reaching a 50% survival when using implant A versus B. A second method to compare two curves is the *log-rank test*. This is one of the most common statistical tests to compare the cumulative survival probability of two groups (e.g., two treatments or two prognostic factors) and is a type of hypothesis testing approach. The test considers the entire distribution of results over the observation or study period, and similar to the application of a t-test or an ANOVA test, it does not adjust for confounders (Chapter 12). In Figure 8.3, let's assume that the p-value is 0.002, which means that the null hypothesis (with a significance level of 0.05)—no difference in survival

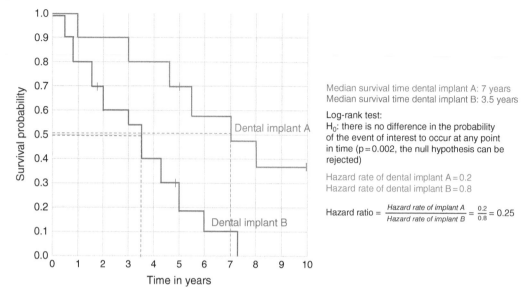

Figure 8.3 Kaplan–Meier curve of a hypothetical study comparing two dental implants and showing median survival time, log rank test, and hazards ratio associated with the outcome of dental implant failure after 10 years follow-up.

probability—can be rejected (Chapter 5). There is a statistically significant difference in the cumulative probability between the group receiving implant A compared to the group receiving implant B. A third method to compare two survival curves is to calculate a per-group *hazard rate* (synonymous with hazard), which is the slope of a survival curve and represents how rapidly subjects are experiencing the event of interest at any point in time. A hazard rate is also defined as the risk of having an event of interest at any particular time point. To compare two hazard rates, a HR (comparing two rates) is calculated, which can be understood as a weighted relative risk accounting for the entire study duration. A HR of to 1.0 means that at any given point, the risk or the probability of experiencing the event of interest (in our example implant failure) is the same for the two groups being compared (implants A and B). A HR below 1.0 means that at any given point, the treatment group (using implant A) has a lower risk or probability of experiencing the event of interest (implant failure) in relation to a comparison group (implant B). A HR above 1.0 means that at any given point, the treatment group (using implant A) has a higher risk or probability for the event (implant failure) to occur in relation to a comparison group (using implant B). In the example in Figure 8.3 the hazard rate for participants in the group receiving dental implant A is 0.2, while implant B it is 0.8 (Appendix 1, Formula 8.2). The calculated HR in this example is 0.25 ($\frac{0.2}{0.8} = 0.25$). This means that at any given time during the follow-up period (10 years), patients receiving implant A were 0.25 (25%) times as likely to experience implant failure by the next time point compared to those receiving implant B. Another way to frame the interpretation of these results is that at any given time during the follow-up period (10 years), patients receiving dental implant A had a 75% reduction in the risk of experiencing implant failure compared to those receiving implant B.

Cox proportional hazard model

The *Cox proportional hazard model*, also called proportional hazard regression, uses a regression approach to determine the association between a time-to-event outcome of interest and one (univariable) or more covariates or predictors (multivariable) (Chapter 11). Among the predictors, investigators may include the variable of interest (e.g., intervention or exposed versus control or nonexposed) and any other variable that can be a potential confounder (e.g., age, sex, socioeconomic status) and requires adjustment or is an effect modifier (Chapter 12). Results from a Cox proportional hazard model optimally include a HR, the 95% confidence interval of the HR (Chapter 6), and a p-value (Chapter 5).

A few additional notes

- While the log-rank test is one of the most popular statistical tests used to compare the cumulative survival probability of two groups, other tests, including the *Wilcoxon test* and the *Peto test,* serve a similar purpose. The main difference is that the latter tests emphasize distances between the curves at the beginning of the curve (early on in the study), whereas the former highlights differences at the end of the curve (later on in the study).
- Some models are based on the assumption that the hazard rates always are proportional among two or more groups under comparison (the *proportional hazard assumption*). One such model is the Cox proportional hazard model, which assumes that the estimated HR is the same at every single point in time and any differences that may be observed are due to *random error*. This assumption will be violated every time the hazard rate for presenting the outcome of interest varies between groups, for example, being low at the beginning of the observation period and much higher by the end. Under such a scenario, the HR is an average of the lower and higher estimates, which makes the final estimate misleading. The proportional hazard assumption is applicable to any variable included in the model.
- Visual and statistical methods allow investigators to determine the validity of the proportional hazard assumption. One simple visual method is to identify whether the two survival curves being evaluated cross each other at the beginning or in the middle of the observation period. If the curves cross each other or lose their parallelism, one concludes that the proportional hazard assumption is not met and the analysis is invalid. However, there is an exception, which corresponds to observing the two curves under evaluation crossing each other by the end of the study when very few participants are left followed up. If this is the case, it is not evidence of a violation of this assumption.

Water slide park and Kaplan–Meier curve interpretation

Water parks have a variety of slides with different colors, lengths, slopes, and age and height requirements. One sunny day you stand atop a platform, with two waterslides stretching out in front of you. The red slide is famous for being steep and fast. You approach the top of the red slide and cannot even see the finish. Next, you observe the blue slide, often the plan B for those scared of the red slide, as it is less steep, meaning a lower speed of descent. In general, why are we more worried about steeper slides than those that decline more gradually? The answer is that if something goes wrong (e.g., getting severely injured), the consequences would be much more severe on steeper than more gradual slides. In other words, the risk of something undesirable happening anywhere throughout the length of a steeper slide is higher the steeper the slide. When comparing two Kaplan–Meier curves representing two treatment options (red and blue survival curves or waterslides), an eyeball comparison of the slope of the curves can give an initial impression of the risk of the outcome or event of interest with one treatment compared to another. The slide's slope represents the hazard rate—the slope of a survival curve—and represents how rapidly subjects present the event of interest over time. In our example, the slope of the slide represents how rapidly subjects go from the top to the bottom of the slide.

Selected readings

Bland JM, Altman DG. The logrank test. *BMJ.* 2004;328:1073.

Bland JM, Altman DG. Survival probabilities (the Kaplan-Meier method). *BMJ.* 1998 Dec 5; 317(7172):1572.

Prinja S, Gupta N, Verma R. Censoring in clinical trials: review of survival analysis techniques. *Indian J Community Med.* 2010 Apr;35(2):217–221.

Schober P, Vetter TR. Survival analysis and interpretation of time-to-event data: the tortoise and the hare. *Anesth Analg.* 2018 Sep;127(3):792–798.

Sedgwick P. Cox proportional hazards regression. *BMJ.* 2013;347:f4919.

Sedgwick P. Hazards and hazard ratios. *BMJ.* 2012;345:e5980.

Sedgwick P. How to read a Kaplan-Meier survival plot. *BMJ.* 2014;349:g5608.

9

Understanding and interpreting a probabilistic-based diagnosis

Treatment decisions should be grounded on an accurate diagnosis. However, the process involved in deciding if a test is needed, interpreting the results, and establishing a diagnosis is fraught with uncertainties. Statistics can quantify and reduce these uncertainties by using a probabilistic-based diagnostic model. Such an approach is based on a progressive sequence that starts with the probability of disease before any examination or testing (*pretest probability*, also known as *prior probability*) to the probability of disease after a clinical workup and testing (*posttest probability*, also known as *posterior probability*) to a final diagnosis. As treatment interventions are always associated with both benefits and harms, being able to determine when the benefits outweigh the harms helps inform treatment decisions. One advantage of using a probabilistic-based approach to guide decision making is the ability to set *clinical thresholds* where the benefit-to-harm ratio has been considered and favors the indication of a test.

Using results from a test can help clarify and quantify the uncertainties in establishing a diagnosis. The ultimate question facing a clinician is, "What does the result mean?" For example, there may be a 10% chance that a person who truly has a disease will get a wrong diagnosis or a negative test result (a false negative result) or a 10% chance that a person without a disease will test positive (a false positive result). Informing a patient that they "probably" or "likely" have or do not have a disease does communicate uncertainty as well as probability. In our example, the 10% quantifies this uncertainty. When interpreting a test result, there are several concepts or measures that can help quantify the uncertainty and the test performance that should be considered: *prevalence, sensitivity, false negative rate* (FNR), *specificity, false positive rate* (FPR), *positive predictive value* (PPV), *negative predictive value* (NPV), *test accuracy, positive likelihood ratio* (LR⁺), and *negative likelihood ratio* (LR⁻) (Table 9.1).

Prevalence is a measure of the presence of disease among a population, usually expressed as a percentage. For example, the prevalence of COVID-19 in a particular population of 10,000 individuals is 3%, which means that there are 300 ($0.03 \times 10,000 = 300$) individuals with COVID-19 and 9,700 ($10,000 - 300 = 9,700$) individuals without COVID-19. All 10,000 individuals were tested for COVID-19 (Table 9.2) (Chapter 15).

Sensitivity

Sensitivity is the probability of a positive test result among all persons with the disease. It is a measure of a test's ability to detect disease correctly when it is present. This is also known as the *true positive rate* (TPR). In our example, if 285 of the 300 individuals with the disease tested positive,

Statistics for Dental Clinicians, First Edition. Michael Glick, Alonso Carrasco-Labra, and Olivia Urquhart.
© 2024 John Wiley & Sons, Inc. Published 2024 by John Wiley & Sons, Inc.

Table 9.1 Overview of test characteristics and test outcomes.

	Disease present	Disease absent		
Test result positive	**True positive (TP)**	**False positive (FP) (type I error)**	**Total positive test results** Σ True positive test result $+$ Σ False positive test result	**Positive predictive value (PPV)** $\dfrac{\Sigma \text{ True positive test result}}{\Sigma \text{ Test result positive}}$
Test result negative	**False negative (FN) (Type II error)**	**True negative (TN)**	**Total negative test results** Σ True negative test result $+$ Σ False negative test result	**Negative predictive value (NPV)** $\dfrac{\Sigma \text{ True negative test result}}{\Sigma \text{ Test result negative}}$
	Total population with the disease Σ TP$+\Sigma$ FN	**Total population without the disease** Σ TN$+\Sigma$ FP	**Total population** Σ TP$+\Sigma$ FN $+$ Σ TN $+\Sigma$ FP	
Positive likelihood ratio (LR$^+$) $\dfrac{\text{TPR}}{\text{FPR}}$	**True positive rate (TPR, sensitivity)** $\dfrac{\Sigma \text{ True positive}}{\Sigma \text{ Disease positive}}$	**False positive rate (FPR, 1−specificity)** $\dfrac{\Sigma \text{ False positive}}{\Sigma \text{ Disease negative}}$	**Accuracy** $\dfrac{\Sigma \text{ TP}+\Sigma \text{ TN}}{\Sigma \text{ Total population}}$	
Negative likelihood ratio (LR$^-$) $\dfrac{\text{FNR}}{\text{TNR}}$	**False negative rate (FNR, 1−sensitivity)** $\dfrac{\Sigma \text{ False negative}}{\Sigma \text{ Disease positive}}$	**True negative rate (TNR, specificity)** $\dfrac{\Sigma \text{ True negative}}{\Sigma \text{ Disease negative}}$		

Table 9.2 True positive, true negative, false positive, and false negative values according to prevalence, sensitivity, and specificity.

	Disease present	Disease absent	Total
Test positive	285 TP	970 FP	1,255
Test negative	15 FN	8,730 TN	8,745
Total	300	9,700	10,000

The result of a hypothetical example where 10,000 individuals with a 3% prevalence of COVID-19 were examined with a test with a sensitivity of 95% and specificity of 90% (Appendix 1, equations 9.1–9.7a).

the sensitivity of the test would be 95% (Appendix 1, Equation 9.1, Table 9.2). Sensitivity can answer the question, "What percentage, or how many, positive test results would we expect among all individuals with the disease?" Sensitivity doesn't convey if a positive test result for an individual patient is a true positive or (TP) a false positive (FP) test result but only suggests the probability of obtaining a TP test result.

The FNR is the probability of a negative test result in a person with the disease. In our example, if 15 of the 300 individuals with the disease tested negative, the FNR is 5% (Appendix 1, Equation 9.2). As a person with the disease can test only negative or positive, the FNR is the difference between all individuals with the disease and the sensitivity (1 − sensitivity = FNR). The FNR can answer the question, "What percentage, or how many, negative test results would we expect among all individuals with the disease?"

Specificity

Specificity is the probability of a negative test result in a person without disease, or a measure of a test's ability to detect the absence of disease when the disease is truly absent. This is also known as the *true negative rate* (TNR). In our example, if 8,730 of the 9,700 individuals without the disease tested negative, which means the specificity of the test is 90% (Appendix 1, Equation 9.3). Specificity can answer the question, "What percentage, or how many, negative test results would we expect among all individuals without the disease?" Specificity doesn't convey if a negative test result for an individual patient is a true negative or a false negative test result but only suggests the probability of obtaining a TN test result.

False positive rate is the probability of a positive test result in a person without the disease. In our example, if 970 of the 9,700 individuals without the disease tested positive, the FPR would be 10% (Appendix 1, Equation 9.4). As a person without the disease can test only negative or positive, the FPR is the difference between all individuals without the disease and the specificity (1 − specificity = FPR). The FPR can answer the question, "What percentage, or how many, positive test results would we expect among all individuals without the disease?"

Positive predictive value

Positive predictive value is the percentage of all TP test results among all positive test results (TP+FP). In our example, the PPV is 22.7% (Appendix 1, Equation 9.5). The PPV can answer the question, "What is the chance (probability) of a positive test result being a TP result?" In our example, a positive test result means that the chance of the individual with a positive test result having the disease is 22.7%. A PPV can be applied to an individual patient and interpreted as a risk for having the disease given a positive test result.

Negative predictive value

Negative predictive value is the percentage of all TN test results among all negative test results (TN+FN). In our example, the NPV is 99.8% (Appendix 1, Equation 9.6). The NPV can answer the question, "What is the chance (probability) of a negative test result being a TN result?" In our example, a negative test result means that the chance of the individual with a negative test result not having the disease is 99.8%. A NPV can be applied to an individual patient and interpreted as a risk for not having the disease given a negative test result.

Test accuracy is the proportion of all true positive test results plus all true negative test results divided by the total number of test results when the test is used in a specified population. In our example, the test accuracy is 90.15% (Appendix 1, Equation 9.7a). Unfortunately, test accuracy does not provide a distinction between FP and FN test results and can sometimes provide a very skewed reflection of a test's ability (Appendix 1, Equation 9.7b).

If a test is needed and if such a test is indicated for the specific disease of interest, a diagnostic or screening test will increase or decrease an estimated probability of the presence or absence of disease beyond what is known before the test is performed. Consider this example: You receive a phone call from a patient, a 65-year-old male, who describes a lesion on the lateral border of his tongue and wants to know what it could be. Without examining the patient, you make a differential diagnosis that includes ulcerative lichen planus and oral squamous cell carcinoma (OSCC). The likelihood of these pathologies can be quantified by knowing the prevalence or incidence of these conditions among 65-year-old males. The prevalence of OSCC or ulcerative lichen planus among a patient population can be used as the probability of a patient's condition before any other information is known. At this stage in the diagnostic process, this is the pretest probability. After a thorough medical history, clinical examination, and test (a biopsy), a definitive diagnosis is made. This is the posttest probability, which could either increase or decrease the probability of the lesion being an OSCC or ulcerative lichen planus. In view of these results, a treatment decision is made.

The pretest probability of disease—in the above scenario, the prevalence—is required to calculate the posttest probability of disease—the pretest probability with the addition of the interpretation of a test result—which is the information needed for any treatment decision. In our example of testing for COVID-19 using a test with a sensitivity of 95%, a specificity of 90%, and a prevalence of 3%, obtaining a positive test result moves diagnostic uncertainty from a pretest probability of having the disease of 3% to a posttest probability—the PPV—of 22.7% (Appendix 1, Equation 9.8a). If the same test is now applied in another city with a higher prevalence, such as 5%, the PPV would have been 33.3% (Appendix 1, Equation 9.8b; Table 9.3). Importantly, if we do not have the prevalence, we will determine our own pretest probability, and if our pretest probability is the same as the prevalence, the posttest probability will be the same.

Table 9.3   Predictive values, prevalences, sensitivities, and specificities.

	Prevalence				
	1%	**3%**	**5%**	**10%**	**20%**
Sensitivity/specificity	Positive predictive value (PPV)/Negative predictive value (NPV)				
80%/80%	3.9%/99.7%	11.0%/99.2%	17.4%/98.7%	30.8%/97.3%	50.0%/94.1%
85%/85%	5.4%/99.8%	14.9%/99.5%	23.0%/99.1%	38.6%/98.1%	58.6%/95.8%
90%/90%	8.3%/99.9%	21.8%/99.7%	32.1%/99.4%	50.0%/98.8%	69.2%/97.3%
95%/95%	16.1%/99.9%	37.0%/99.8%	50.0%/99.7%	67.9%/99.4%	82.6%/98.7%
99%/99%	50.0%/100%	75.4%/100%	83.9 %/99.9%	91.7%/99.9%	96.1%/99.7%

See Disease Screening Interpretation—Penn Dental Medicine (upenn.edu) (https://www.dental.upenn.edu/research/center-for-integrative-global-oral-health/resources/disease-screening-interpretation/).

Likelihood ratios

Likelihood ratios (LRs) differ importantly from PPV and NPV as LRs can be estimated without knowing the prevalence of a disease. If the TPR (sensitivity) and the TNR (specificity) remain the same, the prevalence is irrelevant to estimate LRs. The prevalence will change the TP, FN, TN, and FP cases, but the ratios of the rates (TPR, FNR, TNR, FPR) are not affected by the prevalence. Using LRs provide a great advantage if the interpretation of a test result is conducted among a specific population or subpopulation where the prevalence is unknown. For example, although the prevalence of COVID-19 may be known for New York City (NYC), this prevalence may not be reflected in a particular dentist's patient population, which consists of individuals who couldn't work remotely throughout the COVID-19 pandemic and most probably have a higher COVID-19 prevalence than NYC as a whole. In this type of situation, two pieces of information, the presence or absence of a disease based on a test result, can be combined as a ratio.

The LR is the proportion of test subjects with the disease of interest to the proportion without the disease who have the same test result, respectively. A positive likelihood ratio (LR$^+$) is the odds of disease in a person with a disease and a positive test result in proportion to the odds of a person without the disease and a ***positive test result***. This can also be expressed as the quotient of the sensitivity and 1 − specificity $\left(\dfrac{senitivity}{1-specificity} = LR^+\right)$ (Formula 9.9). In our example, the LR$^+$ is 9.50 (Appendix 1, Equation 9.9). An LR$^+$ can answer the question, "How likely is it, or what are the odds, that a person with a positive test result has the disease?"

A negative likelihood ratio (LR$^-$) is the odds of a disease in a person with a disease and a negative test result in proportion to the odds of a person without the disease and a ***negative test result***. This can also be expressed at the quotient of 1 − sensitivity and specificity $\left(\dfrac{1-senitivity}{specificity} = LR^-\right)$ (Formula 9.10). In our example, the LR$^-$ is 0.06 (Appendix 1, Equation 9.10). An LR$^-$ can answer the question, "How likely is it, or what are the odds, that a person with a negative test result has the disease?"

As the name implies, the LR is a ratio, and thus if the ratio equals 1, it means that there is no difference between the pretest and posttest probability of a particular test result (a positive test result for a LR$^+$ or a negative result for LR$^-$) between individuals with or without the disease of interest (i.e., doesn't inform practice decisions). Both LR$^+$ and LR$^-$ have the probability of disease in the numerator; thus LR > 1 suggests that the particular test result is more likely to occur in an individual with the disease of interest, while LR < 1 suggests that the particular test result is more likely to occur in an individual without the disease of interest. The larger the difference from 1, the higher the likelihood of presence (LR$^+$) or absence (LR$^-$) of disease. In general, LR$^+$ > 10 or LR$^-$ < 0.1 are strongly associated with the presence or absence of disease, or establishing or excluding a diagnosis, respectively (i.e., the test is useful to rule in or rule out presence of disease).

Together, assessing prevalence or incidence of the disease of interest in the population, the result of a medical history workup, and a clinical examination provides an initial or pretest probability for a diagnosis of the disease of interest. The posttest probability is the estimated probability of making a correct final diagnosis.

Two commonly used methods for estimating the posttest probability are the use of a nomogram (Figure 9.1) and the direct calculation of the posttest probability. The calculation is performed in three steps:

1) Transform pretest probability to pretest odds (Appendix 1, Formula 9.11, Table 9.4).
2) Transform pretest odds to posttest odds (Appendix 1, Formula 9.12).
3) Transform posttest odds to posttest probability (Appendix 1, Formula 9.13, Table 9.4).

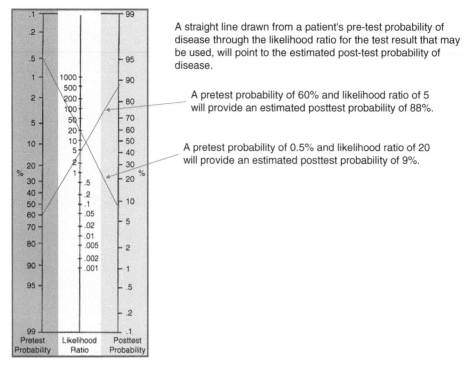

A straight line drawn from a patient's pre-test probability of disease through the likelihood ratio for the test result that may be used, will point to the estimated post-test probability of disease.

A pretest probability of 60% and likelihood ratio of 5 will provide an estimated posttest probability of 88%.

A pretest probability of 0.5% and likelihood ratio of 20 will provide an estimated posttest probability of 9%.

Figure 9.1 Nomogram.

Table 9.4 Converting odds to risk.

Odds	Ratio		Ratio	Probability
9.00	9:1	or	9:1	0.90
4.00	4:1	or	8:2	0.80
2.33	2.33:1	or	7:3	0.70
1.50	1.50:1	or	6:4	0.60
1.00	1:1	or	5:5	0.50
0.67	0.67:1	or	4:6	0.40
0.43	0.43:1	or	3:7	0.30
0.25	0.25:1	or	2:8	0.20
0.11	0.11:1	or	1:9	0.10
0.05	0.05:1	or	5:95	0.05

$$\frac{odds}{odds+1} = probability, \frac{probabilty}{probability-1} = odds$$

When employing the same likelihood ratios to estimate the posttest probability, the pretest probability will be the determining factor for the posttest probability.

Consider this example: A patient presents with multiple ulcerations in the oral cavity. Based on the patient's medical history and clinical examination, the clinician determines that there is a 40% chance (the pretest probability) that the ulcerations are caused by human herpes virus 1

(HSV-1). A test with a sensitivity of 80% and a specificity of 80% is performed and provides a positive result. Based on these parameters, the clinician estimates that the probability of the ulcers being caused by HSV-1 is 72.7% (Appendix 1, Equation 9.11a). If the clinician, based on patient's medical history and clinical examination, would have assigned a pretest probability of 10% for the lesions being caused by cytomegalovirus (CMV), and used the same test as before (i.e., 80% sensitivity and 80% specificity), the posttest probability would have been only 30.7% (Appendix 1, Equation 9.11b).

Using a probabilistic approach to making a diagnosis enables the establishment of a decision-making threshold. Such a threshold can involve whether a treatment is warranted or not and help to determine whether to perform a different workup, including more or different tests, or just to do follow-ups to observe possible progression, remission, or no change of the disease. The threshold bisecting the decision to observe and follow up with the patient or perform a different workup is called the "testing threshold," while that between further diagnostic workup, including testing, and treating the patient is called the "testing-treatment threshold." Starting from a pretest probability that initially warranted the indication of a test, the posttest probability resulting from test application can determine three scenarios: (1) the posttest probability plummets and is lower than the pretest probability to the point that the disease is ruled out, (2) the posttest probability does not change much compared to the pretest probability, warranting further testing, or (3) the posttest probability skyrockets, is much higher than the pretest probability, and crosses the probability threshold (treatment threshold) that warrants implementation of a treatment. There may not be a globally agreed upon level of these thresholds, but they are instead based on a clinician's own experience or clinical judgment, the patient's values or preferences, the availability of specific interventions, and the downstream consequences associated with a test. Any decision on a treatment intervention must also weigh the potential benefits and harms to the patient associated with such a decision. Looking at the example above, where the clinician was faced with making a diagnosis in a patient with oral ulcerations, the clinician decided a priori that a 70% probability or above (i.e., the testing-treatment threshold) of having made the correct diagnosis warranted treatment with an antiviral oral medication. The posttest probability of 72.7% is above this threshold, so the clinician determined that treatment was warranted. The 30.8% posttest probability of the ulcer being caused by CMV would, in the view of this clinician's test-treatment threshold, warrant further testing that could have increased or decreased the posttest probability.

The probabilistic diagnostic process involves four steps:

1) Establishing a pretest probability based on, if known, the prevalence or incidence of the disease of interest, a patient's chief complaint, a patient's medical and dental history, and a physical examination, all of which will lead to a differential diagnosis.
2) Exploring and deciding on a particular test or tests, which includes weighing the benefits and harms to the patient associated with performing the test(s). After deciding which test to use, perform the test.
3) The pretest probability and correct interpretation of the test result(s) to establish a posttest probability of making a correct diagnosis.
4) The posttest probability to make decisions about treatment interventions or further workups and tests.

A probabilistic approach to making a diagnosis will support alternative courses of action after making a differential diagnosis and a tentative (using the treatment/further workup and testing threshold) final diagnosis, and thus reduce the chance of making a misdiagnosis.

Needing a new car with the goal of arriving on time
I usually take my car when going from NYC to Philadelphia. The trip is 105 miles, and a friend of mine estimated that the trip should take an average of 105 minutes. However, with my present very old car, I estimate that the trip will take 120 minutes. However, one day my car was being repaired and I was given a brand-new car as a loaner from the carshop. With this new car, the trip is now estimated to take only 95 minutes.   The average time can be looked upon as an estimated pretest probability. The ability of a car to go faster or slower resembles a likelihood ratio. Which car I drive will affect my posttest probability. The old car has a slower speed (likelihood ratio A) and increases the estimated travel from 105 minutes to 120 minutes (my posttest probability). The loaner has a different speed (likelihood ratio B) and will also affect my posttest probability, reducing the time of travel to an estimated 95 minutes (my new posttest probability). I decided to buy a new car.

Selected readings

Bossuyt PMM. Interesting diagnostic test accuracy studies. *Semin Hematol.* 2008;45:189–195.

Dahm MR, Crock C. Understanding and communicating uncertainty in achieving diagnostic excellence. *JAMA.* 2022;327(12):1127–1128.

Djulbegovic B, van den Ende J, Hamm RM, Mayrhofer T, Hozo I, Pauker SG; International Threshold Working Group (ITWG). When is rational to order a diagnostic test, or prescribe treatment: the threshold model as an explanation of practice variation. *Eur J Clin Invest.* 2015;45(5):485–493.

Glick M, Carrasco-Labra A. Screening testing in health care: getting it right. *J Am Dent Assoc.* 2022;153(4):365–370.

Morgan DJ, Meyer AND, Korenstein D. Improved diagnostic accuracy through probability-based diagnosis. Rockville, MD: Agency for Healthcare Research and Quality; September 2022. AHRQ Publication No. 22-0026-3-EF.

10

Understanding and interpreting a correlation

Correlation and *regression* are two related statistical concepts using the same data points. A correlation estimates the strength and direction of a relationship between a pair of *variables*, whereas a regression expresses the relationship between variables in the form of an equation that can be used to make inferences about the *effect* of an intervention or *exposure* on an *outcome*, as well as prognosis and prediction.

More specifically, a correlation is the extent to which a change in the value on one (sometimes also more than one) variable—the *independent variable*(s)—results in a corresponding (fixed amount) change on a second variable—the *dependent variable*. Understanding and interpreting *regression* analyses will be addressed in Chapter 11.

Pearson product-moment correlation

Measures of association—*absolute risk difference*, *relative risk*, and *odds ratio*—are used for *dichotomous outcomes*, for which there are only two possible options—an *event* either happened or did not (Chapter 2). There are other situations where researchers are interested in quantifying the *association* or correlation between variables (e.g., *risk factors*, *predictor variables*) that are measured using a *continuous* scale (*interval scale* or *ratio scale*) with a *continuous* outcome of interest. Examples of continuous outcomes are decayed, missing, filled teeth (DMFT), clinical attachment level, oral-health-related quality of life, and mouth opening.

The *Pearson product-moment correlation coefficient* (r; sometimes referred to as the *Pearson correlation coefficient* or *Pearson's r*) is one of the most common measures of association used in science to examine linear relationships between continuous variables.

With two continuous variables of interest, a correlation coefficient provides information about whether an association exists and, if so, its strength and direction. The coefficient ranges from –1 through 0 to +1. The strength of a correlation is a unit-free number. The associated plus or minus sign represents the direction of the correlation. When r = 0, no correlation exists, while r values close to –1 or +1 represent a strong correlation. A perfect correlation exists when r = –1 or +1. Thus, r = –0.50 corresponds to the same magnitude of an association as r = +0.5, but these relationships have opposite directions. A negative correlation (or an inverse or indirect relationship) is represented by a minus sign and indicates that as the values for one variable increase, the values for the other decrease, while a positive correlation (or a direct relationship) is represented by a plus sign and indicates that as the values for one variable increase, the values for the other also increases.

Statistics for Dental Clinicians, First Edition. Michael Glick, Alonso Carrasco-Labra, and Olivia Urquhart.
© 2024 John Wiley & Sons, Inc. Published 2024 by John Wiley & Sons, Inc.

These two correlations are symmetrical or bidirectional, where the correlation between variable 1 and variable 2 is the same as the correlation between variable 2 and variable 1 (Figure 10.1).

A *scatterplot* is a graphical representation of the potential association between two *quantitative variables* of interest. The position of a dot on the plot corresponds to a value for an individual or a unit of analysis that represents the magnitude of a dependent variable of interest on the y-axis (vertical axis) and the independent variable of interest on the x-axis (horizontal axis). For example, Figure 10.2 shows a scatterplot of the association between the height (x-axis) and body weight (y-axis) of 18 individuals. For this association r = +0.74, suggesting a strong and direct correlation between the variables. In addition, the figure shows a best-fit straight line, estimated so that the distances of every x value and corresponding y value (x, y) from the observed data to the line are as short as possible. The closer, on average, the x and y values are to this line, the stronger the correlation between them.

The correlation coefficient can also reflect the extent to which a linear component can explain the association between the two variables of interest, where a change in one unit of a continuous independent variable, usually depicted on the x-axis, is associated with a fixed unit of change in the other continuous (dependent) variable of interest, usually depicted on the y-axis. Figure 10.2

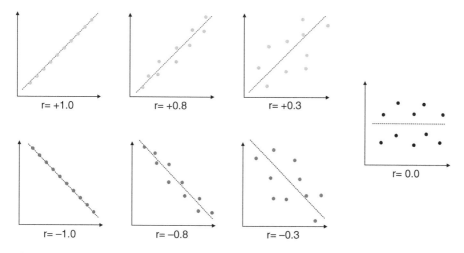

Figure 10.1   Scatterplots illustrating different values of correlation coefficients (r).

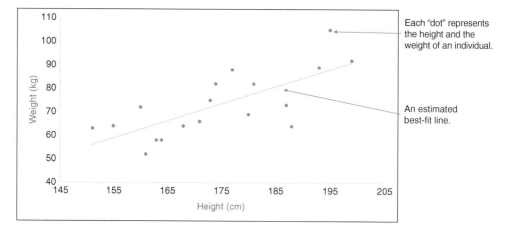

Figure 10.2   Scatterplot displaying the correlation between height and weight for 18 individuals.

illustrates the linear component (line of best fit) for measures of height (x-axis) and weight (y-axis) among 18 individuals. The figure suggests that for every additional centimeter of height, an individual would weigh an additional 0.73 kg (Chapter 11).

Interpretation of Pearson correlation coefficients and coefficient of determination

Correlations focus on the degree of difference rather than similarities among the observed data. Scholars have proposed several approaches to interpret the strength of a correlation, including the use of descriptors like "weak," "strong," or "moderate," which correspond with a value threshold for r. While most scholars agree on what are considered negligible (r<0.1) and very strong (r>0.9) correlations, intermediate values are less consistent (Table 10.1). For example, in 1942 Dean and colleagues published an article in *Public Health Reports* addressing the association between the content of fluoride in parts per million (ppm) contained in the water supply of 21 U.S. cities and the caries experience of children in those communities (Figure 10.3).[1] Using the data set presented in the original study, the correlation coefficient between the two variables is −0.86 (95% confidence interval; −0.94 to −0.67). This correlation is negative, which means that as the fluoride content in the water supply goes up, the magnitude of caries experience in the children goes down, suggesting an inverse relationship between the variables. The value of r = −0.86 is considered a very strong correlation between the variables. Like other measures of association, correlations are also accompanied by their measure of *variability*. The 95% confidence interval around the estimate suggests that the correlation can be as large as −0.94 (very strong, almost close to a perfect negative correlation) or as little as −0.67 (a moderate negative correlation) (Chapter 6). Researchers may fail to report a confidence interval and instead provide a p-value accompanying the correlation coefficient. In this example, the p-value for the correlation between fluoride in the water supply and caries experience is <0.0001. The null hypothesis (H$_0$: r=0) is thus rejected in favor of the alternative hypothesis that the observed correlation coefficient is different from zero. As with any hypothesis-driven significance testing (Chapter 5), rejecting the null hypothesis provides no information about the strength of the association between the variables of interest, nor does it represent a threshold for *clinical significance* (Chapter 20).

Table 10.1 Magnitude of correlation coefficient and interpretation of the strength of association

Observed correlation coefficient	Interpretation of the association
0.0 = |r|	No correlation
0.0 < |r| < 0.2	Very weak correlation
0.2 ≤ |r| < 0.4	Weak correlation
0.4 ≤ |r| < 0.6	Moderately strong correlation
0.6 ≤ |r| < 0.8	Strong correlation
0.8 ≤ |r| < 1.0	Very strong correlation
1.0 = |r|	Perfect correlation

|r|—absolute value of the correlation coefficient.

1 Dean HT, Arnold FA JR, Elvove E. Domestic water and dental caries. *Public Health Rep.* 1942;57:1155–1179.

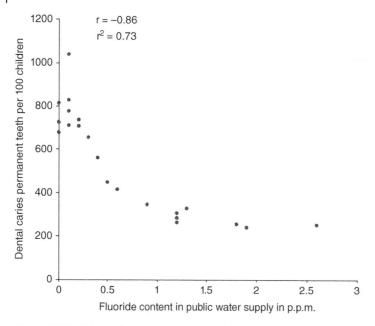

Figure 10.3 Relation between magnitude of dental caries per 100 children (12–14 years old) and the fluoride content in public water supply of 21 cities (blue dots) in 4 states in the United States (n = 7,257 children) in 1940.

Correlations are often used to develop research hypotheses. For example, a hypothesis may be put forth suggesting that a variable X should somehow be related to another variable Y. If a correlational study is performed and an association is found, the finding helps to support the hypothesis.

Although quite informative as a stand-alone value, a correlation coefficient should always be accompanied by a scatterplot. When r = 0, the data points will appear scattered randomly across the plot, and when the value of r is close to +1 or −1, the points will align in a line along the graph. In the example from Dean and colleagues each dot represents a city in the United States (21 dots). The position of each dot in the graph is determined by the concentration of fluoride in the water supply (in ppm) on the x-axis and the frequency of caries experience (caries in permanent teeth over 100 children) on the y-axis (Figure 10.3). A visual inspection of the distribution of dots on the graph supports the information provided by r. There is a relatively tight negative correlation (downward trend) between the variables, with an initial steep slope reaching a possible plateau starting at 1.5 ppm. These observations of potential patterns or distributions are only possible when a scatterplot accompanies the correlation coefficient and better contributes to understanding the phenomenon of interest.

An additional estimate is the *coefficient of determination* (r^2). This coefficient is the square of the correlation coefficient and is interpreted as the proportion of the variance in the dependent variable that is accounted for by the independent variable, under the assumption of a linear relationship. This value ranges from 0 to 1, can be presented as a percentage, and is always a positive number (Figures 10.4, 10.5). In the fluoride-caries study, r = −0.86 and r^2 = 0.73, or 73%. In plain English, this means that approximately 73% of the variability of the caries experience in children's permanent teeth can be explained by the relationship with the concentration of fluoride in the water supply in ppm observed in the 21 U.S. cities. This also means that there is a residual 27% of the variability that remains unexplained by water fluoridation.

Figure 10.4   Representation of two uncorrelated variables, correlation coefficient (r) and coefficient of determination (r²). All of the variance in variables 1 and 2 is independent of one another, represented by the lack of overlap between the squared figures.

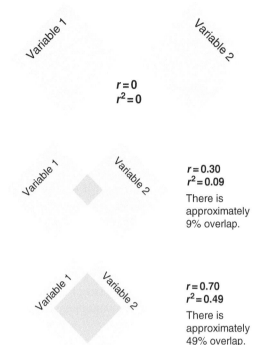

Figure 10.5   Representation of two pairs of correlated variables, correlation coefficient (r), and coefficient of determination (r²). The precise percentage of the shared variance can be determined by squaring the correlation coefficient (r). The squared correlation coefficient (r²) is called the coefficient of determination. The r² magnitude is represented by the degree of overlap between the squared figures. When r² = 0.49, 49% of dependent variable can be explained by the independent variable and 51% is associated with some other variable(s).

Misinterpretation of correlations

A common saying is that "correlation is not causation" (Chapter 12). When a very strong correlation, like the one observed by Dean and colleagues, is found between water fluoridation and caries experience ($r = -0.86$), there are three potential explanations: (1) the presence of classic and straightforward causation, which means that having fluoride in the water supply causes a preventive effect on caries experience in children with no other variables affecting the association; (2) a more complex causation model may exist where water fluoridation and caries experience remain associated, but another variable(s) may reduce or increase the observed level of association; and (3) no causal link between the two variables and the observed correlation may be spurious (see additional information below). These three possible explanations reflect the limited value that correlations offer in establishing causation but also their contribution as hypothesis generators. Remember that correlations are symmetrical or bidirectional, meaning variable 1 is just as likely to precede variable 2 and vice versa. Thus, the cause-effect temporal sequence between the variables and, in turn, causality cannot be established. The presence of a large correlation coefficient does not mean that a causal relationship exists, but such a finding may encourage researchers to further explore such an association using other types of study designs and statistical methods. Another common mistake is extrapolating a correlation to information beyond the data observed in a study. This is addressed in more detail in the chapter addressing regression analysis (Chapter 11). Spurious relationships also exist. A now classic example was published in the *New England Journal of Medicine*.[2] Here the

---

2 Messerli FH. Chocolate consumption, cognitive function, and Nobel laureates. *N Engl J Med.* 2012 Oct 18;367(16):1562–1564.

researcher hypothesized that chocolate has a cognitive benefit and "proved" this by showing a strong and positive correlation between national chocolate consumption and the number of national Nobel laureates.

A few additional notes

- Spearman's rank correlation coefficient (r_s) is used when one or both variables are ordinal, extreme outliers are present, there is a small sample size, or there is no clear linear relationship between the variables (e.g., the dots on a scatterplot are not approximately aligned in a linear formation).
- Spearman's rank correlation coefficient is the nonparametric (statistical methods where there are few or no assumptions about the shape of the distribution or the parameters) version of Pearson's product-moment correlation coefficient and is also called Spearman's ρ (rho).
- Kendall's rank correlation coefficient, also known as Kendall's τ (tau), is an alternative to Spearman's rank correlation that can be used under similar scenarios and lead to comparable inferences about the correlation of the data.
- A phi coefficient (denoted by φ or r_φ) or the mean square contingency coefficient is similar to the Pearson coefficient, but instead of quantifying correlations for continuous variables, the phi coefficient is used for quantifying the correlation between two binary (male/female, yes/no, true/false) variables.

The puppy walk conundrum and the direction of a correlation

Anyone who has walked a puppy on a leash for the first time would understand how much patience is needed to walk a puppy for just a few blocks. A new puppy and its owners go for a walk around the neighborhood for the first time. One of the owners tells his partner, "A friend told me that we can motivate the puppy to walk using treats." So every time the puppy does not want to walk, the owners give the puppy a treat and the walk resumes for a short time. They repeated this action several times on every block during the walk. The owner concluded, "Every time the puppy does not want to walk, we give it a treat, and the problem is solved! It starts walking again! Treats are great motivators" (i.e., treats → walking). If we could read the puppy's mind, it might be thinking, "Every time I want a treat, I stop walking, and I get one! Life is good!" (walking → treats). Both variables, the puppy not walking and the owners offering treats, are highly correlated in the owner's and the puppy's minds. However, no one can determine whether the treats motivate the puppy to walk as puppies cannot speak their minds (direction of a correlation).

Selected readings

Bland JM, Altman DG. Statistics Notes: Correlation, regression, and repeated data. *BMJ.* 1994;308:896.

Cumming G, Calin-Jageman R. Correlation. In: *Introduction to the New Statistics: Estimation, Open Science, and Beyond.* Routledge;2016:293–328.

Guyatt G, Walter S, Shannon H, Cook D, Jaeschke R, Heddle N. Basic statistics for clinicians: 4. Correlation and regression. *CMAJ.* 1995 Feb 15;152(4):497–504.

Hung M, Bounsanga J, Voss MW. Interpretation of correlations in clinical research. *Postgrad Med.* 2017 Nov;129(8):902–906.

Messerli FH. Chocolate consumption, cognitive function, and Nobel laureates. *N Engl J Med.* 2012 Oct 18;367(16):1562–1564.

Sedgwick P. Correlation versus linear regression. *BMJ.* 2013;346:f2686.

Sedgwick P. Spearman's rank correlation coefficient. *BMJ.* 2014;349:g7327.

11

Understanding and interpreting a regression analysis

If two *variables* change in tandem in the same direction (directly or positively) or in different directions (inversely, indirectly, or negatively), they can be considered correlated and the magnitude of this *correlation* can be quantified (e.g., with the *Pearson product-moment correlation coefficient*, Spearman's rank correlation coefficient) (Chapter 10). Regression is an extension of this concept in which an equation or *model* is derived to describe how the expected value of some variable—a *dependent variable*—is related to the values of one or more other *variables—independent variables*. A dependent variable depends on the value of some other variable(s) and is also referred to as an *outcome*, response, or predicted variable. Independent variables can help explain the variability in the values of the dependent variable and are sometimes described as predictors, *exposures*, covariates, or explanatory variables. The terminology used to describe these variables will primarily depend on the purpose of the research, but for simplicity the terms dependent or *outcome variables* and independent variables are used herein.

Regression analysis is a useful tool for researchers who want to go further than just summarizing the frequency of variables in a *sample* (i.e., *descriptive statistics*); regression can also estimate the magnitude of *intervention*/exposure and outcome relationships and make outcome predictions.

Estimation

Clinicians want to know which interventions are the most effective for treating a disease or which behavior changes can prevent future disease. A number of study designs (Chapters 15, 16, 17, and 18) and methodological approaches can answer these questions.

Experimental studies like *randomized controlled trials (RCTs)* are advantageous because study participants are randomized to intervention groups and all known and unknown *prognostic factors* are (or should be) equally distributed between groups (Chapter 18). In a hypothetical RCT, the *mean difference* in caries status (a *continuous variable*) measured using the decayed, missing, and filled teeth (DMFT) *index* at 12 months of follow-up between children who received sealants and those who received fluoride varnish is calculated by taking the difference between the *mean* DMFT at 12 months in each group (Appendix 1, Formula 2.11). Alternatively, this outcome can be measured *dichotomously*, like the presence or absence of caries, and hence the quotient of the *absolute risk* in each group yields an estimate of the *treatment effect* (Appendix 1, Formula 2.4 Chapter 2). In some situations, the RCT design and/or outcome variables are complex and simple methods to calculate measures of association (Appendix 1, Formulas 2.3, 2.4, 2.7, 2.9, 2.11) will produce invalid estimates (also known as spurious estimates) of the treatment effect. Regression equations

Statistics for Dental Clinicians, First Edition. Michael Glick, Alonso Carrasco-Labra, and Olivia Urquhart.
© 2024 John Wiley & Sons, Inc. Published 2024 by John Wiley & Sons, Inc.

provide one way to account for these nuances at the analysis stage to allow for valid inferences about intervention/exposure and outcome relationships.

Data from *observational studies* can pose analytic challenges as there is a need in these types of studies to minimize the impact of *confounders* (i.e., variables that affect both the dependent and independent variables and cause spurious effects) and account for *effect modifiers* (i.e., variables that can explain a difference in a treatment effect across participants' strata between intervention/exposure and outcome; Chapter 12). These complex relationships can be addressed in the design and analysis phases using an appropriate study design and analysis method (i.e., regression analysis).

Prediction

Another practical application of regression is to derive a set of independent variables that best predict a dependent variable. When the goal is to identify a subset of independent variables that can explain a large proportion of the variability or differences in the values of the dependent variable to predict future events, regression analysis is used to make such a prediction.

Irrespective of the research goal (estimation or prediction), the independent and dependent variables in a regression equation can take on many forms (e.g., *continuous, dichotomous, ordinal, time-to-event*) (Chapter 1). The type of data will drive which regression equation to use to analyze observed data.

Linear regression

Linear regression is a subtype of regression analysis that describes the relationship between one or more independent variables and a *continuous* dependent variable. The most rudimentary form of linear regression is *simple linear regression* (SLR), which describes the relationship between two variables. The dependent variable is always continuous, while the independent variable can be continuous or *categorical*. For simplicity, we will address the relationship between two continuous variables (e.g., does an individual's weight (continuous variable 1) depend on their height (continuous variable 2)?) herein, but note that the independent variable can take on other forms (e.g., categorical).

The correlation between two continuous variables can be quantified with a *correlation coefficient*, which indicates the strength and direction of a linear association (Chapter 10). Going one step further, an equation for a line that best fits the data can be estimated—a line of best fit. Suppose a data set contains values for two continuous variables (data pairs) measured for all individuals in the data set, where x is the height variable and y is the body weight variable. A *scatterplot* of these data shows a direct linear correlation between height and weight (Figure 11.1). An equation for the line that best fits these data can be derived from the basic formula of a straight line, a linear formula (Appendix 1, Formula 11.1; Figure 11.2), where y, the value of the dependent variable, equals the sum of the y-intercept (the value of y when x = 0, also referred to as a constant "a") and the slope of the line (the amount that the value of y increases for every one-unit increase in the value of x, "b") (Figure 11.2).

Health care or epidemiological data sets often contain *random variables*. In these data sets every subject is randomly sampled from the population and the value of the dependent variable (e.g., body weight) for an individual may vary, despite the fact that we know the value of the

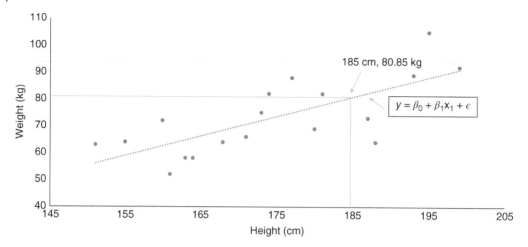

Figure 11.1 Line of best fit and simple linear regression equation for height and weight dataset. A scatterplot depicting measures of 18 persons' height and weight. For the line of best fit, the slope (β_1) is +0.73, the y-intercept (β_0) is -54.2, r is 0.738 and r^2 is 0.545. Interpretation: a strong correlation, a positive direction where for every additional cm of height the person will weigh an additional 0.73 kg. Prediction: What is the estimated average weight for an individual who has a height of 185 cm? $y_i = \beta_0 + \beta_1 x_i$; $\hat{y}_i = -54.2$ + (0.73 x 185 cm) = 80.85 kg

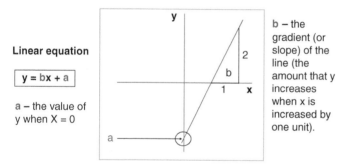

Figure 11.2 Components of a linear equation "a" and "b" are regression coefficients. For example, a slope of 2 means that every 1-unit change along the x-axis yields a 2-unit change along the y-axis.

independent variable (e.g., height). A prediction is not always perfect as there may be other variables not included in the equation that may influence the value of the dependent variable. This variability can be incorporated into the linear equation as a *random error* term or residual term (ε in Appendix 1, Formula 11.2). Thus, similar to a linear equation, in SLR, for a given set of observed data pairs, the average value of the dependent variable (*y* in Appendix 1, Formula 11.2) equals the sum of the *regression coefficients* of x, which are the estimates of the slope (β_1 in Appendix 1, Formula 11.2), and the y-intercept (β_0 in Appendix 1, Formula 11.2) and a random error term (residual term, ε, in Appendix 1, Formula 11.2) representing the variability in y for every randomly selected individual in the population. The regression coefficient for the slope corresponds to how much the dependent variable changes for every one-unit change in the independent variable. A positive number indicates a direct relationship between the variables (when one variable increases, the other variable increases), a negative number an inverse relationship (when one variable decreases, the other variable decreases). The sign of the regression coefficient for the slope has an analogous interpretation with pairwise correlation—where a positive slope corresponds to a positive r (i.e., correlation coefficient), a negative slope corresponds to a negative r, and a slope equal to 0 is equivalent to no correlation (r = 0). Also, the mean of y, given a particular value of x, can be estimated using an SLR equation. In the height and weight example, a regression coefficient of +0.73 means that for every 1 cm increase in height, weight is expected to increase, on average, by 0.73 kg (Figure 11.1).

With regression coefficient estimates from an SLR equation, the average value of a dependent variable can be estimated for a given value of the independent variable. For example, the average weight of someone who is 185 cm is predicted to be 80.85 kg (Appendix 1, Equation 11.1, Figure 11.1). A confidence interval for this mean can also be estimated.

Another useful value that can be derived from fitting data with an SLR equation is the *coefficient of determination*, typically denoted as r^2 (Chapter 10). The coefficient of determination can take on a value from 0 to 1 and is defined as the proportion of variation in the dependent variable that can be explained by the independent variable, in other words, how well the independent variable helps explain the values of the dependent variable (Figure 11.1).

Multiple (or multivariable) linear (MLR) regression

MLR is similar to SLR in the sense that the dependent variable is continuous, with the only difference being the number of independent variables included in the equation. In contrast to SLR, where one independent variable attempts to explain the variability in the dependent variable, in MLR the variability can be explained with two or more explanatory variables (explanatory variable is another term used synonymously with independent variable). The independent variables can again be continuous or categorical.

In MLR regression coefficients are estimated for each independent variable. The value for each regression coefficient corresponds to the estimated change in the dependent variable for a one-unit change in the independent variable holding the rest of the independent variables constant. MLR is typically superior to SLR because it considers many factors that may affect the relationship or that may be useful in predicting the dependent variable. When the effect of an independent variable on a dependent variable is hypothesized to be different depending on a particular value of another independent variable (e.g., diabetes status (yes/no), public insurance status (yes/no), etc.), effect modification may be present. *Interaction* terms can be included in an MLR model (Chapter 12) to explore effect modification. As in SLR, the value of a dependent variable can be predicted from the best set of independent variables. Further, the coefficient of determination (R^2; this time, the R is capitalized because there are multiple independent variables) describes the proportion of variability in the dependent variable that can be described when all of the independent variables are considered together. The larger the R^2, the better the model is at predicting the dependent variable.

Logistic regression

Epidemiologists are interested in knowing if an exposure is associated with an increased risk of developing an outcome. When the outcome is dichotomous, as in the case of periodontal disease status (disease = yes or no), *logistic regression* can help predict the probability or risk of an outcome and estimate the association between an exposure/intervention and a categorical outcome.

Predicting risk and odds

A logistic model is an equation that allows for the estimation of the probability or risk of experiencing an event for an outcome (Appendix 1, Formula 11.3), proving useful when dealing with a dichotomous dependent variables. For example, in the context of a cohort study (Chapter 17), logistic regression is useful for predicting the relative or absolute difference in the risk of developing an outcome between two groups. Furthermore, the mathematical properties of a logistic model allow for the model to be written in an equivalent way called the "logit form." This mathematically equivalent form results in an expression representing the natural logarithm (ln) of the *odds* of experiencing an event for an outcome or the dependent variable (Appendix 1, Formula 11.4). Exponentiating the constant, e, by this expression will result in an estimate of the odds of an outcome (Appendix 1, Formula 11.5). This allows for the estimation of an individual's odds (Appendix 1, Formula 11.5) and risk or probability (Appendix 1, Formula 9.13) of experiencing an event for an outcome (Chapter 2), given a set of independent variables or risk factors with logistic regression. Just like in linear regression, regression coefficients are estimated for each independent variable included in the equation.

A hypothetical example: predicting risk and odds of an outcome

Consider a data set from a cohort study (Chapter 17) that contains the periodontal disease status (yes/no) for all individuals (dependent variable) and potential *risk factors* for the disease, including current smoking status (yes/no), alcohol use (yes/no), history of cardiovascular disease (yes/no), diabetes (yes/no), and toothbrushing (yes/no) for each individual in the cohort (independent variables). After fitting the data with a logistic equation, the regression coefficients for the independent variables smoking status, alcohol use, cardiovascular disease, and diabetes are all positive numbers, meaning they contribute to or increase the risk of periodontal disease. On the other hand, the regression coefficient for toothbrushing is negative, meaning that toothbrushing is protective against periodontal disease or decreases the risk of periodontal disease (Table 11.1).

In this cohort, if an individual (person 1) was a smoker, was a user of alcohol, had cardiovascular disease, had diabetes, and brushed their teeth, using the estimates for the regression coefficients from Table 11.1, their estimated odds of periodontal disease would be 53.52 (Appendix 1, Equation 11.2). The risk (probability) of disease can be estimated by transforming odds to risk; thus, with odds of 53.52, the risk of having periodontal disease is 98.16% (Appendix 1, Equation

Table 11.1 Regression coefficient estimates from a dataset used to derive a logistic regression model.

Independent variable	Regression coefficient estimate
Constant (intercept)	−3.12
Smoking	3.21
Alcohol use	1.68
Cardiovascular disease (CVD)	1.62
Diabetes	2.92
Toothbrushing	−2.33

Person 1: smoking = yes, alcohol use = yes, cardiovascular disease = yes, diabetes = yes toothbrushing = yes.
Person 2: smoking = no, alcohol use = no, cardiovascular disease = yes, diabetes = no, toothbrushing = yes.

11.3) Alternatively, the risk of the outcome in an individual can be derived directly from the logistic model (Appendix 1, Formula 11.3). Another individual (person 2) also had cardiovascular disease and brushed their teeth but neither smoked nor used alcohol and did not have diabetes. Without these additional risk factors (smoking, alcohol use, and diabetes), again, using the estimates for the regression coefficients in Table 11.1, this person's estimated odds of periodontal disease would be 0.022 (Appendix 1, Equation 11.2) and their corresponding risk would be 2.15% (Appendix 1, Equation 11.3). This comparison of the risk of periodontal disease in person 1 and person 2, derived from the coefficient estimates from a logistic regression equation, tells us that smoking, alcohol use, and diabetes contribute to the risk of periodontal disease much more than cardiovascular disease and toothbrushing do.

Estimating odds ratios

The logistic model's computational strength lies in its ability to deal with data from a range of observational study types (e.g., cohort, case-control, and cross-sectional studies) as the regression coefficients from a logistic regression equation can be utilized to estimate odds ratios (ORs).

A hypothetical example—estimating an odds ratio

In a hypothetical case-control study (Chapter 16) of children with and without birth defects (dichotomous dependent variable), values for the mothers' folic acid supplementation during the first month of pregnancy (dichotomous independent variable) were collected. The regression coefficient for the exposure of interest derived from a logistic regression equation can be used to estimate a crude OR and 95% confidence interval for the association between a mother's intake of folic acid supplements and birth defects status of their child (Appendix 1, Formula 11.6). If the regression coefficient for folic acid supplementation is –0.5, then the OR would be 0.61 (Appendix 1, Equation 11.5). The OR derived from a logistic regression equation fit with this data set with just two variables (one dependent variable and one independent variable—*simple logistic regression*) will be identical to the OR derived from the classic contingency table (i.e., 2 × 2 table) approach to calculate an OR (Appendix 1, Formula 2.7 and Formula 2.9)—a *crude effect estimate* of the OR. It is called a crude OR because there is only one independent variable in the logistic regression equation (i.e., folic acid).

In the context of observational study designs (e.g., cohort, case-control, cross-sectional studies), rarely can an association between one independent variable (e.g., folic acid consumption) and an outcome (e.g., birth defects status) be estimated without considering potential confounders or accounting for variables that may modify the effect (effect modifiers) between the exposure and outcome of interest (Chapter 12). Once potential confounders and effect modifiers are identified, they can be included as independent variables in the logistic regression model. The final model with multiple independent variables (i.e., exposures, confounders, effect modifiers) is called *a multivariable or multiple logistic regression* model.

In the same way that a crude OR was derived from the logistic regression model with just one independent variable, the regression coefficient estimates from a multivariable logistic regression model can be used to derive an *adjusted effect estimate* for the measure of association—one that controls for confounders (Chapter 12). In other words, given that all confounders are held constant, the study was conducted according to appropriate methodological standards, and the appropriate statistical model was used, the adjusted OR estimate is the *unbiased estimate* of the association between an exposure and an outcome. Further, if a variable is determined to be an effect modifier, an OR can be estimated for each level of the variable or subgroup.

Nonindependence of observations

An assumption so far in all the aforementioned regression models, is that all observations for the dependent variables are independent from one another. In cluster RCTs or longitudinal studies (Chapters 17 and 18) this assumption does not hold true. If the unit of randomization in a cluster RCT is a classroom, the students in that classroom would have a series of common individual features that would not make the outcome measures or observations independent from one another. In a longitudinal study, enrolled individuals may have multiple visits at which an outcome is measured. The data collected from all of these visits are not independent observations, but they are correlated. Regression models such as generalized estimating equations or generalized linear mixed models (or random effects or hierarchical models) can account for the nonindependence of the data.

Building a regression model

Building a model is more of an art form than an exact science. More than one valid model may appropriately fit the data. The first step in building a model is hypothesizing a relationship between the dependent and independent variable(s) for the data and then choosing an appropriate regression equation. Next, investigators verify any assumptions that the model employs. When deciding on which independent variables to include in the model, the goal (estimation vs. prediction) of the analysis will be the driving force. There are methods to choose independent variables to include in the model for when prediction or when estimation is the goal. Using the wrong method can lead to incorrect inferences. There are also methods for ensuring that the chosen model best fits the data (i.e., *goodness of fit tests*) and checking to see if independent variables are not contributing the same information (*collinearity*), both of which contribute to the ultimate goal of deriving a final model.

A few additional notes

- The *ordinary least squares method* is a common technique to derive regression coefficients in linear regression. The difference in the actual data points from a sample and the estimated fitted values (i.e., the line of best fit) is called the sample residuals (Figure 11.3). Ordinary least squares is a way of estimating regression coefficients to minimize these sample residuals or the distance between the estimated line of best fit and the sample data.
- Sometimes regression coefficients are *standardized* so they can be compared in a given study or across studies and are denoted by the symbol "β" to distinguish them from unstandardized regression coefficients which are denoted by the symbol "b".
- Hypothesis testing and SLR: With the SLR line of best fit estimate, the question of whether X helps at all in predicting Y under the assumption of a linear relationship between the variables can be answered. This is equivalent to asking whether the correlation between X and Y

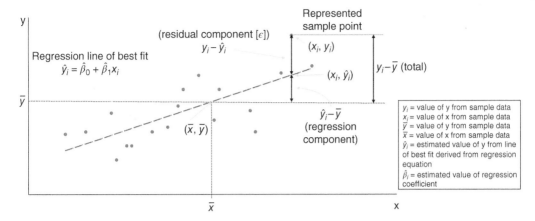

Figure 11.3 Simple linear regression line. The difference in the sample data points and the line of best fit (yi–ŷi) is called the residual component. The difference in the value of y for the line of best fit and the estimated mean of y from the sample data (ŷi–ȳ), is called the regression component. The method of least squares, minimizes the residual component in the estimation of the regression equation (i.e., line of best fit).

is not equal to 0. The null hypothesis for this question would be whether the regression coefficient for the slope and intercept is equal to 0. With the regression coefficients for the slope and intercept and their associated standard errors (Chapter 4), a test statistic (under the *t-distribution*) and corresponding p-value and 95% confidence interval can be derived to test this hypothesis. Another way to test this hypothesis is with an *F-statistic*, which is simply the square of the t-statistic. The corresponding p-values for these tests will be equivalent. Analogously, in MLR an F-statistic and corresponding p-value will provide insights into whether the independent variables considered together significantly explain the variation in the dependent variable.

- Predictions and SLR: Suppose a more specific question is of interest beyond the average value of the dependent variable given some value of an independent variable. This more specific question could be, "If a person from the target population walks in the door and their height is 185 cm, what will the value of their weight be?" Their weight, on average, will be the same as the estimated mean value of weight calculated in Figure 11.1 (80.5 kg), but a *prediction interval* instead of a confidence interval around the estimate for their weight is derived. On top of random variability, the variability of the person walking in the door is incorporated into the prediction interval. Prediction intervals are inherently wider than 95% CIs because of this extra variability.

- A logistic regression model is derived from a logistic function. The possible values for the logistic function range from 0 to 1, proving useful for modeling epidemiological data because the risk or probability (Chapter 2) of disease also ranges from 0 to 1.

- In logistic regression, as in linear regression, hypothesis tests can assess if the derived OR is statistically significantly different from 1 (Table 2.2). Common statistical tests include the Wald test and likelihood ratio test, each having advantages under certain conditions, but both generally resulting in the same conclusion with large samples.

- Statistical tests for interaction and modeling strategies can help determine if the independent variables (i.e., potential confounders and effect modifiers) included in a logistic regression equation are modifying or confounding the intervention/exposure and outcome relationship the researcher is attempting to estimate, and if they should stay in the model.

- Special cases of logistic regression: Sometimes a categorical outcome may not be dichotomous and instead may take on values for more than two levels. Special types of logistic regression can be used to model both *nominal* and *ordinal* outcome data (Chapter 1). Polytomous logistic regression was developed for the former and the proportional odds model for the latter. In case-control studies, cases and controls are often matched on potential confounders. An approach called conditional logistic regression can account for matching in the analysis.
- Other types of regression: When "time-to-event" or "survival" data are obtained from a study, a specialized regression model called Cox regression is appropriate to fit the data and estimate a hazard ratio (Chapter 8). When the dependent variable is a count (e.g., the number of daily car crashes in North Carolina), Poisson regression is an appropriate equation to use.

Prediction with multiple linear regression

Tom is hosting a birthday party for his wife Mindy and has invited her entire family for the affair. For dessert, Tom would like to surprise Mindy and make her grandmother's secret extra-fudgy brownie recipe. He locates the recipe but is horrified to see that a lot of the ingredient quantities and instructions are smudged. Tom did not plan very well, and the party begins in three hours. With key parts of the recipe missing, he must decide if he should attempt to make the brownies or just go and buy some at the store. He knows that if he makes them, they must be fudgy, as Mindy's family despises cakey brownies. In fact, Mindy's family has a Fudgirometer that measures the fudginess of brownies on a continuous scale, with scores between 75 and 90 being deemed the ideal fudginess.

Tom is happy to have found some eggs, butter, canola oil, flour, cocoa powder, vanilla extract, chocolate chips, and sugar in his kitchen. He also locates both a silicone and an aluminum baking pan. Can Tom make fudgy brownies with the ingredients and materials he has on hand? He does a quick search on the internet and finds an interesting article. It turns out that Betty Crocker already knows the secret to making fudgy brownies, after taking a road trip across the United States and sampling brownies for their fudginess with the Fudgirometer from bakeries along the way. Betty was lucky to be able to get all of the recipes and fit a linear regression equation with the information from the recipes that best predicted the fudginess of the brownies. It turns out the type of egg (1 = yolks, 0 = full egg), type of fat (1 = butter, 0 = avocado), baking tray (1 = silicone, 0 = aluminum), and oven temperature (0–500°F) matter the most when predicting brownie fudginess. In other words, together these recipe attributes explain a lot of the variability in brownie fudginess (i.e., large R^2). The regression coefficient for a silicon baking pan is negative, meaning that the use of this pan compared to aluminum will contribute to a decrease in the fudginess score. On the contrary, the regression coefficients for the type of fat, egg, and oven temperature are positive, meaning that egg yolk, butter, and increased temperature contribute to an increased fudginess score.

Tom had an egg yolk, two sticks of butter, and an aluminum baking pan and was able to decipher from the faded recipe that the oven should be preheated to 375°F. He plugged in these values into the regression equation and was relieved to find out that on average his brownies should score 85 on the fudginess scale! Tom decided to make the brownies with these ingredients and what he could salvage from the recipe, and the day was saved!

Estimating exposure/intervention and outcome relationships

Mindy's family loved Tom's recipes so much (dare they say, even better than Grandma's) that they asked him to make them for every family gathering. Mindy's family is so large that Tom was making the brownies every few weeks. He was becoming concerned about all of the butter in the brownies and its effects on the health of his beloved in-laws. Considering heart disease runs in Mindy's family, Tom was especially concerned. What he really wanted to know is if a diet high in saturated fat (i.e., some exposure) will increase the risk for heart disease (i.e., some outcome) in the future. If it will increase their risk too much, Tom will need to consider swapping out the butter in his recipe for something lower in fat.

If Tom had a data set containing information about individuals' dietary fat intake and whether or not they developed heart disease he could make inferences about whether dietary fat intake has an effect on getting heart disease. Of course there may be other factors like age and socioeconomic status that could muddle (i.e., confound) this relationship, or factors like presence or absence of a certain gene that could make this relationship different (i.e., modify it). Lucky for Tom, he found a paper on the internet that used a regression model to estimate this relationship, where the independent variables were dietary fat intake (main exposure of interest), age and socioeconomic status (potential confounders), and presence of some gene (potential effect modifier). Now, he can use the equation to estimate the association between the main exposure, dietary fat intake (high or low), and the risk of heart disease, all while getting rid of these things that may muddle the relationship (i.e., confounders like socioeconomic status) and incorporating aspects that may make the relationship different (effect modifiers like the presence or absence of a gene). After fitting the data with a regression model, the paper concluded that dietary fat is associated with a 200% increased odds of developing heart disease. Looks like Tom will be swapping out that butter for avocado.

Selected readings

Ali P, Younas A. Understanding and interpreting regression analysis. *Evid Based Nurs.* 2021;24(4):116–118.

Bender R. Introduction to the use of regression models in epidemiology. *Methods Mol Biol.* 2009;471:179–195.

Bland JM, Altman DG. Correlation, regression, and repeated data. *BMJ.* 1994;308(6933):896. doi:10.1136/bmj.308.6933.896.

Guyatt G, Walter S, Shannon H, Cook D, Jaeschke R, Heddle N. Basic statistics for clinicians: 4. Correlation and regression. *CMAJ.* 1995;152(4):497–504.

Harris JK. Primer on binary logistic regression. *Fam Med Community Health.* 2021;9(Suppl 1):e001290. doi:10.1136/fmch-2021-001290.

Sedgwick P. Logistic regression. *BMJ.* 2013;347:e4488.

Sedgwick P. Multiple regression. *BMJ.* 2013;347:e4373.

Sedgwick P. Simple linear regression. *BMJ.* 2013;346:e2340.

12

Understanding and interpreting confounding and effect modification

Conducting clinical studies using an appropriate and fair control group is essential in *etiological* and *prognostic studies* as well as in *comparative effectiveness research*. All these types of studies address the extent to which an *exposure* (e.g., therapeutic or preventive *intervention*, a *risk factor*) is associated with an *outcome* (e.g., *binary* or *continuous variable*). An *exposure* is a factor or a type of determinant that can be beneficial (i.e., *protective factor*) or harmful (i.e., risk factor) depending on its expected effect on an outcome of interest. For example, people largely believe that chicken soup helps cure the common cold. If one consumes chicken soup at the early stages of the onset of illness, in most cases, the cold will go away within 72 hours. But what if one skips the soup altogether? Many interesting questions emerge when determining the potential causal effect of chicken soup in curing the common cold after three days. To answer this question, researchers benefit from using a *control group* and working under a what-if scenario or a *counterfactual framework*.

Counterfactual framework and causal reasoning

The concept of counterfactuals can be understood by conducting a thought experiment. Going back to the question above, a researcher is interested in investigating the *association* between consuming chicken soup (the exposure) and experiencing clinical recovery at 72 hours (the outcome). Many factors could potentially explain why people feel recovered on the third day; however, the investigator is exclusively interested in the role that the chicken soup might play in that outcome, independent of any other potential factor. The ideal way to answer this question would be the following: First, the investigator recruits participants at *risk* of getting a common cold who will wait for the initial symptoms to appear. Then, the participants will consume the chicken soup, followed by a measure of the occurrence or risk for the outcome after 72 hours (recovery from the common cold). Second, and as part of our thought experiment, the investigator benefits from owning a time machine and invites the same participants to go back in time to the very moment that the symptoms of the common cold started to manifest. The investigator instructs the participants to do everything as before, with one important exception: no chicken soup consumption. The time machine would help to determine whether the chicken soup is solely responsible for the recovery. Time travel allows for keeping constant all the variables that might influence the outcome (e.g., immunological state, hydration levels, virus subtype, unknown yet relevant individual characteristics). Time

Statistics for Dental Clinicians, First Edition. Michael Glick, Alonso Carrasco-Labra, and Olivia Urquhart.
© 2024 John Wiley & Sons, Inc. Published 2024 by John Wiley & Sons, Inc.

traveling is still a figment of the imagination, and so clearly the second scenario is fictional. The first scenario is real and can be observed (based on real data), while the second is fictitious (cannot be directly measured and is "counter to the facts") and corresponds to the counter-factual scenario.

After performing the thought experiment study, the investigator will be able to determine the risk of recovering from the common cold given that no soup was consumed, which corresponds to the risk in the unexposed group or *baseline risk* (also called *background risk*) or the risk independent from the chicken soup. The risk in the exposed group includes two components: (1) the baseline risk of recovery independent of the chicken soup and (2) the additional risk for recovery attributed to the soup. If the soup provides no additional benefit, the *absolute risk* in the group having and not having the soup will be equal (Chapter 2).

Causal inference and confounding bias

An exposure has a causal effect on an outcome if the occurrence of such outcome in an individual exposed is different from the observed effect in another unexposed individual. This is an oversimplification, as in most cases the observed outcome is linked to several intrinsic and extrinsic factors. These factors can play different roles in a causal model. For example, for an adverse outcome, an exposure that reduces the probability of such an outcome happening would be a protective factor. An exposure increasing the probability of an undesirable event to occur would be a risk factor. Notice that here the word "risk" refers not to the probability of an outcome but rather that the factor may produce an unfavorable event. Thus, *causal inference* aims to disentangle these complex connections between exposures and outcomes, including the different relationships among them, with the purpose of predicting an exposure-outcome association or relationship.

A confounding variable or *confounder* is a factor that distorts or muddies the association between an exposure and an outcome. There are key criteria that a variable should meet to be considered a confounder. The confounder, first, should affect both the exposure and the outcome of interest and, second, should not be affected by the exposure or the outcome (Table 12.1). For example, one can observe that living in Florida (i.e., the exposure) can be associated with a higher risk of having Alzheimer's disease (i.e., the outcome). However, before accepting this statement, it is necessary to explore to what extent the association is biased by confounding: could there be anything but living in Florida that would influence having Alzheimer's disease (Figure 12.1)?

In this case, older adults looking for warmer weather often move to Florida and older adults, are diagnosed with Alzheimer's disease more frequently than other age groups. The apparent association between living in Florida and having Alzheimer's is confounded by age. With age as a confounding variable, the potential proposed association between living in Florida and having Alzheimer's disease is invalid.

Figure 12.2 illustrates a hypothetical study to determine an exposure-outcome association between two groups of participants—group 1 and group 2. The exposure increases the absolute risk of experiencing the outcome by 10% (additional risk due to the exposure). The figure shows that regardless of whether group 1 or group 2 is assigned as exposed or unexposed, the expected baseline risks of experiencing the outcome are the same (i.e., group 1 and 2 = 30%). In addition, the estimates calculated to determine the presence of an association are the same in scenario 1 and scenario 2. This concept is described in epidemiology as the *exchangeability of baseline risks,* which indicates an unconfounded association. In contrast, Figure 12.3 illustrates the opposite situation. The exposure still increases the absolute risk of experiencing the outcome by 10% (additional risk due to the

Table 12.1 Bias (systematic error), confounding, and effect modification and their implications in research and practice.

Concept	Research implications	Practical implications
Bias (systematic error)	Limitations in methods to select participants, collect and analyze data, or report study findings resulting in a deviation or distortion from the truth.	Studies at high risk of bias tend to distort effect estimates (i.e., under- or overestimating the effect), which can result in the misguided application of research findings to patient care.
Confounding (confounding variable or confounder)	An identified association between exposure and outcome is distorted because a third lurking variable is associated with both the exposure and the outcome, but it is not causal by itself (type of bias).	When investigators do not control for or fail to adjust for confounding properly, their results are at high risk of bias. This lowers the credibility of the study findings, which can result in the misguided application of research findings to patient care.
Effect modification (subgroup effect)	An identified association between exposure and outcome differs across the levels of a third variable (e.g., older vs. younger adults) that modifies the observed effect (not a type of bias).	If a subgroup claim prove trustworthy, investigators should report effect estimates separately for each subgroup. Clinicians should indicate the intervention of interest differently across subgroups. If clinicians ignore a trustworthy subgroup effect, they will observe heterogeneous treatment responses among patients (highly effective in some, highly ineffective in others).

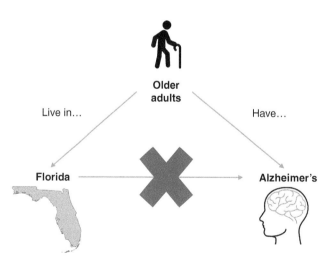

Figure 12.1 Hypothetical example of a confounder. The apparent association between living in Florida and having Alzheimer's is confounded by age. Age is a confounding variable.

exposure); however, the baseline risks of experiencing the outcome between group 1 and group 2 are not the same (i.e., group 1 = 40%; group 2 = 30%). Thus, depending on whether group 1 or group 2 is assigned to be exposed or unexposed, we would observe different results. The measures of association in scenario 1 suggest that there may be no exposure-outcome association, while the estimates in scenario 2 suggest the presence of an association. This means that there is a lack of exchangeability of baseline risks—a confounded association.

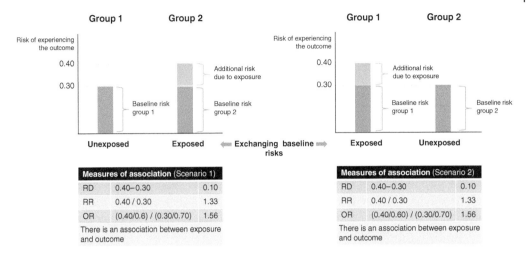

Figure 12.2 Example of exchangeability of baseline risks—unconfounded association. RD: risk difference; RR: relative risk (risk ratio); OR: odds ratio. Note how in scenario 1, group 1 is the unexposed group, and group 2 is the exposed group. This is switched in scenario 2. The values of RD, RR, and OR did not change after switching the groups. Therefore, there is an unconfounded association between exposure and outcome.

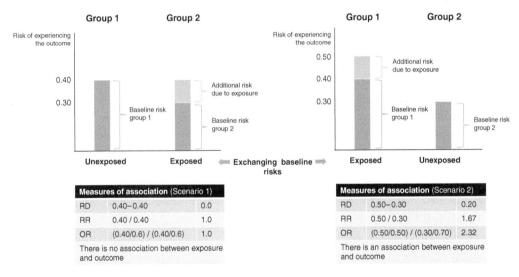

Figure 12.3 Example of lack of exchangeability of baseline risks—confounded association. RD: risk difference; RR: relative risk (risk ratio); OR: odds ratio. In scenario 1, where no associations were found, i.e., RD=0, RR=1.0, OR=1.0, we cannot know if the reason is because of differences in the baseline risks or the exposure has no impact on the outcome. In scenario 2, where associations were found, i.e., RD≠0, RR≠1.0, OR≠1.0, we cannot know if the reason is because of differences in the baseline risks or the exposure has an impact on the outcome.

Strategies to deal with confounding in the study design phase

Researchers dealing with causal inference dedicate efforts to minimizing the effect of confounding. In the early stages of a study, investigators and other subject-matter experts propose a causal diagram (e.g., *directed acyclic graphs* (DAGs)) that represents the underpinning causal theory. This diagram provides a hypothetical explanation of how the exposure affects the outcome and other variables that may influence or be affected by the exposure and outcome. The resulting causal model is essential to determine study participants' selection and identify variables (e.g., confounding variables) that should be measured and accounted for later in the statistical analysis (Box).

1. Randomization

In a randomized controlled trial (Chapter 18), allocating participants to study arms at random allows investigators to create similar or comparable groups regarding known and unknown *prognostic factors*. When appropriately implemented, the *randomization* process creates exchangeable groups, which means that the baseline risk or the event rate for the outcome of interest in either of the groups would be similar if no exposure occurred (Figure 12.2). Thus, if any difference in an outcome is observed between the groups and the influence of other biases is minimized with a methodologically sound study design, such a difference can be attributed to the exposure (i.e., intervention of interest).

2. Specification

A specification or *restriction* strategy utilizes the study eligibility criteria to exclude participants with the confounding variable. For example, when studying the relationship between oral bacteria count (exposure) and surgical site infection after a third molar extraction (outcome), the presence of periodontal disease could be a confounder in this association. Investigators using specification could decide to restrict participants with a history of or active periodontal disease from entering the study, eliminating the potential confounding effect of the disease on the association. This simple and efficient way to deal with confounding variables is not without limitations. Disregarding participants having active periodontal disease from the study limits the *generalizability* or *applicability* of the results. If the study found that there is no association between bacterial count (exposure) and surgical site infection after third molar extraction (outcome), it may have observed an association in participants with active periodontal disease (this phenomenon is called *effect modification* and will be discussed later in this chapter). Since the investigators restricted the eligibility criteria to include only people without active periodontal disease, they will not be able to explore disease's role in the association.

3. Matching

In *matching*, investigators select cases and controls (*case-control study*) or exposed and unexposed (*cohort study*) individuals with similar attributes or levels of the confounding variable. For example, investigators conducting an *observational study* are interested in determining a possible association between being exposed to treatment A versus treatment B, where variable C is a confounder. In participants exposed to treatment A, the frequency of the confounding variable is 67% (4/6), compared to 20% (4/20) in the group exposed to treatment B. These groups are not comparable, and if an exposure-outcome association is identified, investigators can be fooled by the different distribution of the confounding variable between the groups (Figure 12.4a). To avoid finding a *spurious association*, investigators can implement matching by finding an individual in the group exposed to treatment A who matches the values or features of the confounding variable in the group exposed to treatment B. After applying a matching strategy, both groups have a similar frequency of the confounding variable (67% or 4/6) (Figure 12.4b).

Treatment A
67% Confounding variable

Treatment B
20% Confounding variable

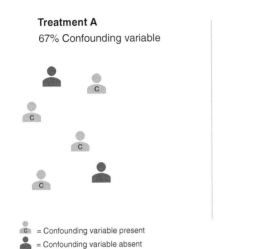
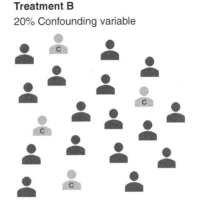

= Confounding variable present
= Confounding variable absent

Figure 12.4a Matching: participants exposed to treatment A and B with dissimilar distributions of a confounding variable.

Treatment A   Confounding variable   **Treatment B**
67%   67%

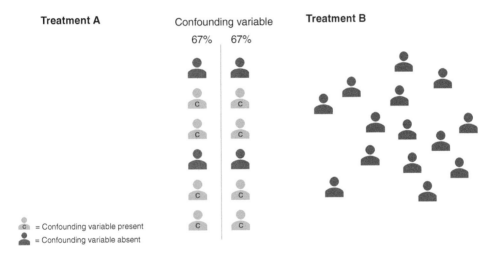

= Confounding variable present
= Confounding variable absent

Figure 12.4b Matching: participants exposed to treatment A and B with similar distribution of a confounding variable after matching. Participants matched according to a confounding variable (vertical line). Participants on the right side who received treatment B did not match with participants on the left side who received treatment A and are excluded from the analysis.

Matching is an effective way to control for confounding variables that are constitutional to an individual (e.g., age, gender). Matching can also facilitate controlling for confounders that are difficult to measure. For example, by matching twins or siblings on factors such as habits, diet, and genetics, confounders can be accounted for at an individual level. By matching study centers on factors such as culture, habits, geography, and treatment modalities, confounders can be accounted for at a cluster level (Chapter 16).

Matching, however, also has some drawbacks. If investigators in a study want to match four or five confounding variables, identifying suitable controls for the cases may be a difficult and time-consuming task. A second limitation is that, as with other strategies to deal with confounding in the design phase, matching is irreversible, and limits further investigation of the effect of the matched variable on the outcome. Third, participants with no matching pair can no longer be part of the study and should be excluded, increasing inefficiencies. Another limitation when using matching is the possibility that the causal model informing the study suggested that a variable is a confounder when in reality that is not the case. In this situation, if the variable remains associated with the exposure while it is not related to the outcome (failing to meet the criteria for a confounder), the study power would be reduced by making the cases and controls more similar, resulting in *overmatching*.

Strategies to deal with confounding in the analysis phase

1. Stratification

Stratification, although implemented at the analysis level, shares commonalities with specification (or restriction) and matching. The goal of stratification is to ensure that the groups under comparison, either cases or controls in a case-control study or exposed and unexposed groups in a cohort study, exhibit similar levels of the confounding variables. This strategy is also used in randomized controlled trials (Chapter 18). To implement a stratified analysis, investigators separate the study participants into small subgroups or strata according to a particular characteristic. For example, a sample can be stratified according to age, socioeconomic status, or any risk factor that can function as a confounding variable for an exposure-outcome. One advantage of stratification is that because it is applied at the analysis level, it provides high flexibility to the investigators to reorganize the data set as needed, a benefit that other strategies, like specification and matching, do not offer. One limitation when using stratification is that investigators need to account or control for several potential variables at a time, which tends to dilute the sample size and overall study power—a function of the number of strata in the analysis (Chapter 7).

2. Propensity score

Investigators can estimate the probability for each individual patient to receive an intervention or treatment of interest given their specific level of prognostic factors. This estimate is called a *propensity score* (also known as propensity-score matching or propensity-score adjustment). De novo collected observational data or existing clinical records are unavoidably affected by *confounding by indication*. This type of confounding occurs because clinicians defining a treatment plan conduct a careful examination of patients' characteristics and prognostic factors. Then, the treatment plan is designed to optimize health care outcomes and prognosis based on the factors. This differential assignment of patients to receive different interventions in clinical practice is highly desirable, as optimizing prognosis is essential in health care. However, the patients who receive a particular treatment tend to be systematically different from those who do not receive that same treatment.

Figure 12.5 depicts a hypothetical observational study using existing medical records that aims to determine the effect of antibiotic prophylaxis prior to a surgical tooth extraction. Patient 1 is a young (1% chance of receiving prophylaxis) female (2% chance of receiving prophylaxis) who does not present with any comorbidities (2% chance of receiving prophylaxis) and has excellent oral hygiene (5% chance of receiving prophylaxis). Based on her prognostic factors, she has a 10% chance of receiving antibiotic prophylaxis after surgical tooth extraction. Patient 2 is an older adult (30% chance of receiving prophylaxis) male (5% chance of receiving prophylaxis) with several comorbidities and polypharmacy (40% chance of receiving prophylaxis) and poor oral hygiene (8% chance of receiving prophylaxis). His probability to receive antibiotic prophylaxis before a surgical tooth extraction, given

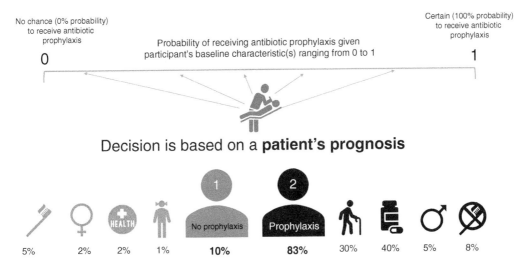

Figure 12.5 Propensity score in two patients undergoing a surgical tooth extraction and indication for antibiotic prophylaxis.

his prognostic factors, is 83%. Instead of adjusting for every individual prognostic factor, investigators can use the propensity scores (10% and 83%, respectively) of patients 1 and 2 to account for all factors at once. This score can be included as a predictor in a multivariable regression model (Chapter 11) or can be used as a tool to choose matched pairs emulating a typical matching approach.

Using the propensity score has advantages. It is an efficient way to adjust for multiple confounding variables simultaneously without the impact on power and precision of other strategies such as stratification. Another benefit is that when defining the confounding variables to control for, it is more straightforward to determine why clinicians indicate a treatment based on a patient's characteristics (i.e., prognostic factors) than to design a theoretical causal model and identify potential confounding variables affecting the exposure-outcome association. The propensity score also has limitations. As with many other methods, the score cannot account for unknown and unmeasured confounding variables, which would remain as residual confounding in the study. Another limitation is that no inferences can be made regarding variables included in the score.

3. Traditional regression modeling

Multivariable regression techniques allow investigators to adjust for several potential confounders at once, where each confounding variable is included as an independent variable (Chapter 11). The purpose of this approach is to produce an estimate of the outcome of interest that is independent of or controlled for measured confounding variables. As with all approaches to adjust for confounding at the analysis stage, regression modeling provides flexibility and is reversible (e.g., in the case that hypothesized confounders included in the regression model do not seem to confound the association). Another limitation specific to regression modeling is that the model is as effective at controlling for confounding as the data fit the confounder-outcome relationship.

After finding evidence of the presence of an association between an exposure and an outcome, investigators should investigate whether such an association is due to the presence of confounding. If the association disappears after adjusting for potential confounders, such an association was likely spurious. Investigators can also explore the extent to which the association differs or remains strong according to levels of a third variable of interest—an effect modifier.

Effect modification

Causal inference is often simplified as the presence of a single exposure (risk or prognostic factor) and its effect on an outcome. This framework, however, is an oversimplification of reality. Rather, many exposures and risk or prognostic factors interact among themselves with different intensities to result in the observation of an outcome. *Effect modification* or *interaction*, or *subgroup effect*, is verified when the association between an exposure and an outcome of interest is affected or modified by a third variable—the modifier (Table 12.1). Figure 12.6 presents three scenarios, with each of them including the results of the administration of an intervention (exposure of interest) and the effect on an outcome of interest among older and young adults (age as a potential *effect modifier*). In scenario 1, the relative effect of the intervention is the same between the old and the young (relative risk = 0.5), which suggests that age is not an effect modifier. When observing the baseline risk (control event rate) in the old versus the young, the old have twice the risk of experiencing the outcome (40%) compared to the young (20%), suggesting that age is a prognostic factor. In scenario 2, the relative risk differs between the old and the young, suggesting that age is an effect modifier for the association between the exposure (intervention) and outcome, with an effect on the old (relative risk = 0.5) and no effect on the young (relative risk = 1.0). In this scenario, however, age is not a prognostic factor as the baseline risk (control event rate) in the old is the same as in the young (20%). In scenario 3, age is both a prognostic factor and an effect modifier. The implication of scenario 3 is that investigators will need to document and report that the intervention may have an important effect on the old but not the young. From a research perspective, exploring effect modification allows disentangling an exposure-outcome association and increases the study's precision by identifying groups that may respond differently to the exposure. From a practical standpoint, the reporting of credible effect modification helps clinicians to identify patient groups that would benefit more or less from an intervention, improving the personalized indication of preventive or therapeutic interventions.

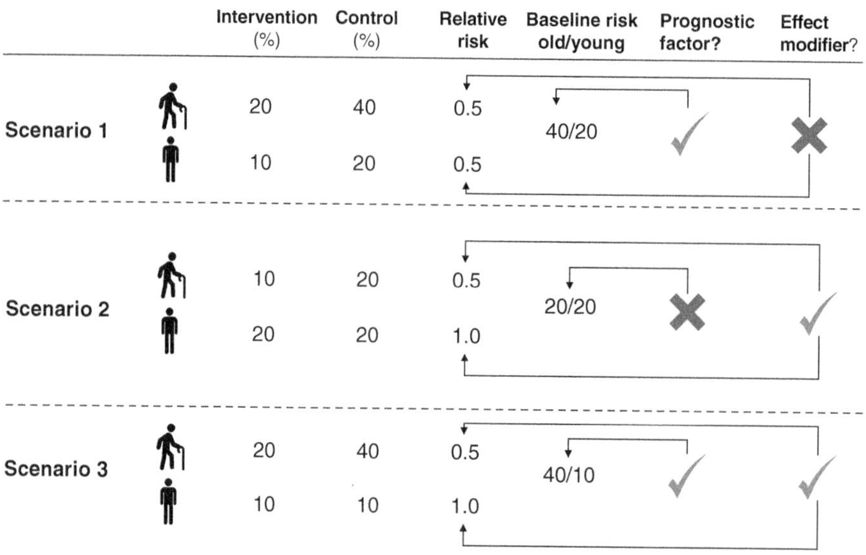

		Intervention (%)	Control (%)	Relative risk	Baseline risk old/young	Prognostic factor?	Effect modifier?
Scenario 1	old	20	40	0.5	40/20	✓	✗
	young	10	20	0.5			
Scenario 2	old	10	20	0.5	20/20	✗	✓
	young	20	20	1.0			
Scenario 3	old	20	40	0.5	40/10	✓	✓
	young	10	10	1.0			

Figure 12.6 Distinction between an effect modifier and a prognostic factor. Three scenarios presenting event rates among older and younger adults exposed to an intervention or a control, and the corresponding relative risk and baseline risk comparison.

A few additional notes

- Possible confounders for the association between sugar consumption (exposure) and early childhood caries (outcome) might include socioeconomic status, parents' caries experience, accessibility to dental care, oral hygiene habits, exposure to fluoride, and level of urbanization of the area of residence. If three strata per confounding variable are suggested, investigators will need to deal with more than 729 strata (3^6, where 3 is the number of levels of each confounding variable and 6 is the total number of confounding variables in the analysis).
- A disadvantage of specification is that it limits the pool of eligible participants, which can impact recruitment efforts and be a threat to reaching the optimal sample size (Chapter 7).
- Remain skeptical of claims of effect modification. It is common to see no real differences across subgroups of patients, but the play of chance is often the reason for investigators to report a subgroup effect. Even if a subgroup effect does not exist, conducting a study testing a large number of subgroup hypotheses could result in a misleading claim of a subgroup effect (type I error).

Box. A hypothetical example of the use of a directed acyclic graph (DAG) to study causal inference

A *directed acyclic graph* (DAG) is a visualization tool that represents the relationships among variables in a causal model. It is the first step in the design of a study aiming to provide evidence of the association between one or more exposures and an outcome of interest. The configuration of a DAG is informed by clinical expertise and the scientific literature, in particular, the evidence on the relative effects—e.g., relative risk, odds ratio—reflected by links connecting exposures (risk or prognostic factors) and an outcome using unidirectional arrows. For example, A → B means that the investigators propose that A (the exposure or predictor) causes B (the outcome).

Figure 12.7a shows a hypothetical DAG constructed to assess the association between high bacterial count and the occurrence of alveolar osteitis after tooth extraction. The orange arrow

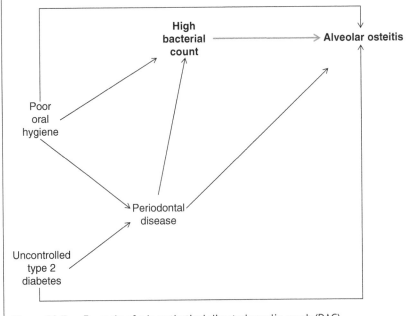

Figure 12.7a Example of a hypothetical directed acyclic graph (DAG).

represents the proposed causal link. In addition, with input from experts in the field and the available evidence, other variables have been proposed that may influence this association: poor oral hygiene, periodontal disease, and uncontrolled type 2 diabetes. The arrows represent the hypothesized associations among variables. After a model is in place, investigators need to identify confounding variables that may mislead the exposure-outcome association. To achieve this, investigators identify every possible alternative pathway that connects the exposure with the outcome that is not part of the direct pathway from exposure to outcome (orange arrow). These pathways are called *backdoor pathways* (sometimes also called confounding pathways). In Figure 12.7b, we are able to identify five backdoor pathways, represented by red, green, blue, black, and purple dotted lines. For example, high bacterial count (the exposure) can be connected with alveolar osteitis through an alternative backdoor pathway via "poor oral hygiene". Consider these lines as pipes or paths that interconnect the exposure and outcome through the variables in the DAG. Notice that these backdoor pathways do not have arrows, as the causal inference information can go in any direction and, in this figure, is currently open.

The next step is to try to block these backdoor pathways in an efficient manner, so the only way that exposure and outcome can be linked is through the causal pathway of interest (e.g., high bacterial count → alveolar osteitis). Adjusting or controlling for a variable (potential confounding) in an open backdoor pathway closes that pathway. For example, Figure 12.7c shows that controlling or adjusting for the variable "poor oral hygiene" blocks the blue, green, and black dotted backdoor pathways. In addition, controlling for "periodontal disease" blocks the red and purple dotted lines. This means that in this DAG "poor oral hygiene" and "periodontal disease" are confounding variables, should be measured as the study is conducted, and should be included in the multivariable regression model to determine if they are actually confounding the effect.

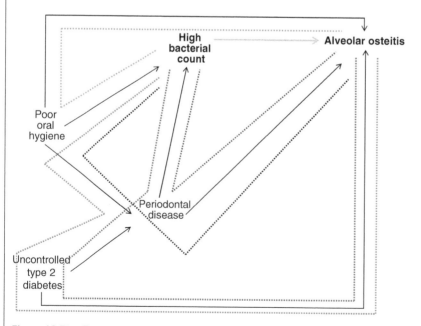

Figure 12.7b Example of a hypothetical directed acyclic graph (DAG) and potential pathways linking variables.

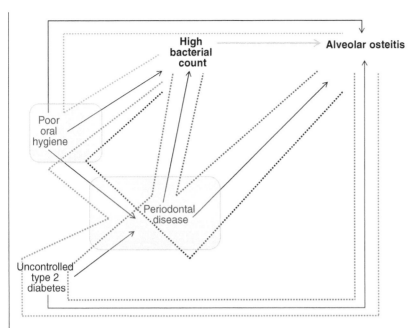

Figure 12.7c Example of a hypothetical directed acyclic graph (DAG) and potential confounding variables to control for in the analysis phase.

Selected readings

Agoritsas T, Merglen A, Shah ND, O'Donnell M, Guyatt GH. Adjusted analyses in studies addressing therapy and harm: users' guides to the medical literature. *JAMA.* 2017 Feb 21;317(7):748–759.

Bours MJL. A nontechnical explanation of the counterfactual definition of confounding. *J Clin Epidemiol.* 2020 May;121:91–100.

Morabia A. History of the modern epidemiological concept of confounding. *J Epidemiol Community Health.* 2011 Apr;65(4):297–300.

Newman TB, Browner WS. Estimating causal effects using observational studies. In: Browner WS, Newman TB, Cummings SR, Grady DG, Huang AJ, Kanaya AM, Pletcher MJ, eds. Designing Clinical Research. 5th ed. Wolters Kluwer; 2023.

Schandelmaier S, Briel M, Varadhan R, et al. Development of the Instrument to assess the Credibility of Effect Modification Analyses (ICEMAN) in randomized controlled trials and meta-analyses. *CMAJ.* 2020 Aug;192(32):E901–E906.

VanderWeele TJ, Shpitser I. On the definition of a confounder. *Ann Stat.* 2013 Feb;41(1):196–220.

Vetter TR, Mascha EJ. Bias, confounding, and interaction: lions and tigers, and bears, oh my! *Anesth Analg.* 2017 Sep;125(3):1042–1048.

13

Understanding and interpreting bias

The term *bias* is colloquially used when one's prejudiced opinion or judgment favors or opposes an issue or motive. Thus, a biased position or statement is different and deviates from an objective judgment or an actual reflection of the "truth." Bias in the context of research has many similarities with this colloquial understanding. Clinicians examining the scientific literature will inevitably find instances where study results are closer to the truth (*accuracy*) or further from the truth (less accurate). Distinguishing each of these occurrences—an essential skill set to inform evidence-based clinical practice—requires an understanding of bias and its implications for creating an appropriate study design and minimizing misrepresentation of the results.

Random error versus systematic error (bias)

In a hypothetical study, a group of investigators aimed to determine the average body weight of the U.S. male adult (aged 20 and over) population. Using calibrated scales, the researchers randomly chose a street corner in New York City and measured the weight of the first 20 male individuals (Sample 1) who, by chance, were passing by. The first estimation of the average, based on Sample 1, was 150 lbs. Intuitively, this value did not seem to be a credible result. Thus, the investigators decided to conduct more measurements. In the second round, they went to the same street corner and used the same scales to measure the body weight of 100 male individuals (Sample 2). This time, the calculated average was 165 lbs. Although this estimate seemed more credible, the researchers decided to increase their sample size again and measured the body weight of 1,000 male subjects at the same street corner (Sample 3). In this third round, the average was 190 lbs., a figure closer to the actual average body weight of the U.S. male adult population—200 lbs. (Figure 13.1).[1] This hypothetical study illustrates the impact of *random error* on the uncertainty around an estimate. Just by chance, a certain group of adult males whose body weight was further away from the average, happened to be passing by during the first measurement, which resulted in an estimate far from the truth (150 lbs. is 50 lbs. from the true mean). As more observations were included and with increased sample sizes, the researchers obtained estimates closer to the true national average, 35 lbs. from the true estimate in Sample 2 and only 10 lbs. off in Sample 3. Sample 1 had a large amount of random error, which was reduced progressively as more people were included (Samples 2 and 3) (Chapter 6).

---

1 The body weight of the U.S. male adult population as reported by the U.S. National Center for Health Statistics.

Statistics for Dental Clinicians, First Edition. Michael Glick, Alonso Carrasco-Labra, and Olivia Urquhart.
© 2024 John Wiley & Sons, Inc. Published 2024 by John Wiley & Sons, Inc.

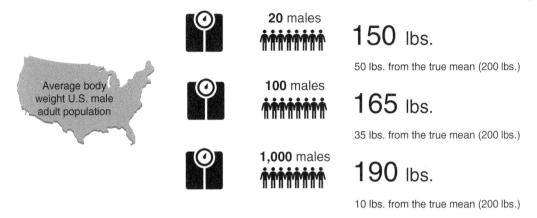

Figure 13.1 Hypothetical scenario of a study measuring the average body weight of the U.S. male adult population among 20, 100, and 1,000 individuals using calibrated scales.

If in the same hypothetical scenario as above the researchers hadn't used appropriately calibrated scales, the results would have been further away from the national average. As an example, the investigators conducted the same three rounds of measures on the same groups of people (i.e., 20, 100, and 1,000 individuals) to determine the average body weight of the U.S. male adult population. But the scales, exposed to the inclement weather for several days, were damaged and provided distorted measures, which resulted in every assessment underestimating the male body weight by 9 lbs. (Figure 13.2). Such *systematic error*, also known as *bias*, leads to inaccurate study results that do not reflect the truth and can lead to an over- or underestimation of a true effect. The use of the word "bias" in the biomedical literature always refers to a systematic error. Unlike issues of random error, an increase in *sample size* alone, say from 20 to 100 to 1,000, cannot solve bias (Figure 13.3).

What does it really mean?

Researchers attempt to minimize random error and biases differently. To diminish random error, they can conduct a *power* analysis to determine an appropriate sample size that will enable them to detect a difference, if present, between treatments under evaluation (Chapter 7). They can also

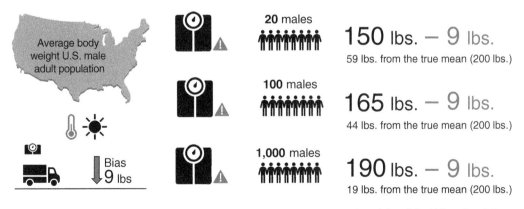

Figure 13.2 Hypothetical scenario of a study measuring the average body weight of the U.S. male adult population among 20, 100, and 1,000 individuals using biased scales.

Random error

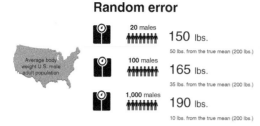

As sample sizes increase, the measures get closer to the "true" average body weight of the U.S. male adult population.

Systematic error (bias)

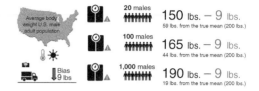

As sample sizes increase, the systematic error in this example (–9 lbs.) remains unrelated to the sample size.

Figure 13.3 Hypothetical scenario of a study measuring the average body weight of the U.S. male adult population among 20, 100, and 1,000 individuals to compare the impact of sample size (number of observations) on random error and systematic error (bias).

construct confidence intervals around their estimates, where narrow intervals reflect less random error and more *precision* and are thus more informative than wide intervals (Chapter 6).

To minimize bias, investigators can implement several methodological strategies, such as selecting an appropriate study design and addressing specific biases inherent to the chosen design (Chapters 15, 16, 17, and 18). The key take-home message is not to confuse issues of bias or accuracy with issues of random error or precision.

There is extensive empirical evidence supporting the view that not addressing different elements when planning a study, including an appropriate study design, how the study is conducted, how the data are analyzed, and how findings are reported, can result in bias. Biases affecting a study have two characteristics: a direction (i.e., underestimating or overestimating an effect) and a magnitude (i.e., trivial or small versus large or substantial). The impact of a particular methodological limitation in two study designs that answer a similar clinical question may differ. For example, one study design may underestimate a *treatment effect*, while another study design may overestimate the same effect. It is impossible to fully ascertain the direction and magnitude of bias in an individual study; only a judgment of the risk of a study being affected by bias is possible.

Distinguishing risk of bias, methodological quality, and reporting quality

Risk of bias, *methodological quality*, and *reporting quality* are often used interchangeably, and although they may be related, these three concepts have different definitions and practical implications. Risk of bias is a judgment of the potential for study results to deviate from the truth due to limitations in the design. This concept differs from methodological quality, which refers to the extent to which the investigators conducted their research to the highest possible standards. However, bias may be present even when a study was conducted according to the highest possible methodological and reporting standards. (i.e., a study with high methodological quality can still be considered at high risk of bias).

For example, a hypothetical study assesses the effect of two different surgical closing techniques on the *outcome* of mouth opening restriction following the removal of impacted mandibular third molars. The different techniques cannot be hidden from the surgeons or researchers in charge of the study, not allowing for *blinding* (Chapter 18). This issue reduces the trial's methodological quality, but the objective clinical measurement—mouth opening restriction—has a low chance of being influenced by awareness of which surgical closing technique was used. Thus, not being able to blind the surgeons or the researchers could only influences the risk of bias minimally. Hence, there is either no or low concerns of bias for this outcome in the context of this study.

Reporting quality, a fundamental element for translating research into practice, is defined as the comprehensiveness and appropriateness of the description of what was done, found, and concluded in a study. Reporting quality is directly related to risk of bias as any assessment of the latter requires an optimal description of the methodological strategies planned and implemented by the investigators. Poor reporting may result in a lack of relevant information to conduct a risk of bias assessment, threatening the trustworthiness of the results. To ensure reporting quality across a variety of designs, the research community conducts extensive consensus exercises for the purpose of agreeing on a standard that includes all necessary items for effective reporting. The Enhancing the Quality and Transparency of Health Research (EQUATOR) network and its platform is the primary source of reporting checklists, cataloged by study design (Table 13.1).[2]

Assessing risk of bias in primary studies

A number of bias assessment checklists are available (Table 13.1) and can be applied to each study outcome or the entire study. Regardless of the design (e.g., randomized controlled trial, cohort study, case-control study) assessed by a particular checklist, there are overarching principles applicable to all analytical study designs:

1) *Selection bias*—Distortion in a measure of association or treatment effect arising from the procedures to identify individuals to enter a study or to be included in the study analysis. *Randomization* is a commonly used strategy to help minimize selection bias when enrolling participants. *Attrition bias* is a type of selection bias resulting from participants lost to follow-up as a study is conducted. Sending reminders and providing participants with incentives to remain in the study are some of the efforts implemented to reduce attrition bias.

2) *Performance* and *measurement bias*—Distortion in the study results due to dissimilar management (performance) of groups under comparison as a study is conducted or a systematic difference in the procedures used to determine (measure) the outcomes. Blinding is frequently used to reduce the impact of performance and measurement bias.

These overarching types of biases take different shapes and gain complexity depending on the study. This is the reason for conducting a targeted risk of bias assessment according to the study design (Table 13.1). These checklists contain questions that allow users to examine whether a specific bias and its underlying operating mechanism are present in a study. It is tempting to simplify assessment results into a single score that reflects the overall risk of bias across domains. However, this approach disregards the fact that domains of bias in a checklist have varying importance. Specific aspects of the study that affect risk of bias include the nature of the outcome measures (e.g., objective or subjective outcomes) and the severity of methodological flaws. The most accepted approach is to avoid single scores and rather present a judgment of the risk of bias that considers each domain, such as selection, attrition, performance, and measurement biases, and more.

---

2 See www.equator-network.org.

Table 13.1 Checklists for risk of bias assessment tools and reporting standards according to study design and type of clinical question.

Study Design	Risk of Bias Assessment tool	Reporting Standard
Clinical practice guidelines	AGREE II (Appraisal of Guidelines Research & Evaluation II) https://www.agreetrust.org/agree-ii/	AGREE (Appraisal of Guidelines Research & Evaluation) Reporting Checklist https://www.agreetrust.org/resource-centre/agree-reporting-checklist/
Systematic reviews of intervention	ROBIS (Risk of Bias in Systematic Reviews) http://www.bristol.ac.uk/media-library/sites/social-community-medicine/robis/robisguidancedocument.pdf AMSTAR (A Measurement Tool to Assess Systematic Reviews) http://www.amstar.ca/	PRISMA (Preferred Reporting Items for Systematic Reviews and Meta-Analyses) https://www.equator-network.org/reporting-guidelines/prisma/Systematic%20reviews
Systematic reviews of diagnostic test accuracy and prognosis	ROBIS (Risk of Bias in Systematic Reviews) http://www.bristol.ac.uk/media-library/sites/social-community-medicine/robis/robisguidancedocument.pdf	PRISMA-DTA (Preferred Reporting Items for Systematic Reviews and Meta-Analyses— Extension for Diagnostic Test Accuracy Studies) http://www.equator-network.org/reporting-guidelines/prisma-dta/
Randomized controlled trials	Cochrane Risk of Bias Tool for Individually-Randomized Parallel-Group Trials (RoB 2) https://sites.google.com/site/riskofbiastool/welcome/rob-2-0-tool Effective Practice and Organization of Care (EPOC) RoB Tool http://epoc.cochrane.org/resources/epoc-resources-review-authors Cochrane Risk of Bias Tool for Cluster Randomized Trials (RoB 2) https://sites.google.com/site/riskofbiastool/welcome/rob-2-0-tool/rob-2-for-cluster-randomized-trials Cochrane Risk of Bias Tool for Crossover Trials (RoB 2) https://sites.google.com/site/riskofbiastool/welcome/rob-2-0-tool/rob-2-for-crossover-trials	CONSORT (Consolidated Standards of Reporting Trials) http://www.equator-network.org/reporting-guidelines/consort/

Table 13.1 (Continued)

Study Design		Risk of Bias Assessment tool	Reporting Standard
Nonrandomized controlled trials		Cochrane ROBINS-I (Risk of Bias in Non-randomized Studies of Intervention) https://sites.google.com/site/riskofbiastool/welcome/home?authuser=0 GRACE checklist (Good Research for Comparative Effectiveness for Observational Studies) https://www.graceprinciples.org Effective Practice and Organization of Care (EPOC) RoB Tool http://epoc.cochrane.org/resources/epoc-resources-review-authors Cochrane ROBINS-E (Risk of Bias in Non-randomized Studies of Exposure) https://sites.google.com/site/riskofbiastool/welcome/robins-e-tool?authuser=0	TREND (Transparent Reporting of Evaluations with Non-randomized Designs) https://www.cdc.gov/trendstatement/index.html
All observational studies	Cohort studies	Cochrane ROBINS-I (Risk of Bias in Non-randomized Studies of Intervention) https://sites.google.com/site/riskofbiastool/welcome/home Effective Practice and Organization of Care (EPOC) RoB Tool (for studies with a control group) http://epoc.cochrane.org/resources/epoc-resources-review-authors NOS (The Newcastle-Ottawa Scale) http://www.ohri.ca/programs/clinical_epidemiology/nosgen.pdf	STROBE (Strengthening the Reporting of Observational Studies in Epidemiology) http://www.equator-network.org/reporting-guidelines/strobe/
	Case-control studies	NOS (The Newcastle-Ottawa Scale) http://www.ohri.ca/programs/clinical_epidemiology/nosgen.pdf Effective Practice and Organization of Care (EPOC) RoB Tool http://epoc.cochrane.org/resources/epoc-resources-review-authors	
	Cross-sectional studies	Joanna Briggs (JBI) Checklist for Cross Sectional Studies https://jbi.global/sites/default/files/2019-05/JBI_Critical_Appraisal-Checklist_for_Analytical_Cross_Sectional_Studies2017_0.pdf AXIS (Appraisal Tool for Cross-Sectional Studies) http://bmjopen.bmj.com/content/6/12/e011458 Joanna Briggs (JBI) Checklist for Prevalence Studies https://jbi.global/sites/default/files/2019-05/JBI_Critical_Appraisal-Checklist_for_Prevalence_Studies2017_0.pdf	

Table 13.1   (Continued)

Study Design		Risk of Bias Assessment tool	Reporting Standard
	Diagnostic test accuracy studies	QUADAS-2 (Quality Assessment of Diagnostic Accuracy Studies) https://www.bristol.ac.uk/population-health-sciences/projects/quadas/quadas-2/	STARD (Standards for Reporting of Diagnostic Accuracy Studies) http://www.equator-network.org/repciling-guidelines/stard/
	Prognostic studies	QUIPS (Quality In Prognosis Studies) Checklist http://methods.cochrane.org/sites/methods.cochrane.org.prognosis/files/uploads/QUIPS%20tool.pdf	TRIPOD (Transparent Reporting of a Multivariable Prediction Model for Individual Prognosis or Diagnosis) https://www.tripod-statement.org/resources/

A few additional notes

- The assessment of the risk of bias using available checklists is often restricted to methodological and statistical aspects.
- A subtle source of bias is referred to as *selective outcome reporting*, which occurs when researchers deviate from the original protocol by omitting outcomes from the final report with the purpose of making the intervention look more favorable than if the entire efficacy and safety outcomes were disclosed. This is also known as cherry-picking the results.
- *Conflict of interest*, a special type of bias, emerges when the judgment of the researchers regarding their primary interest—conducting and reporting sound clinical research—is influenced by a second competing interest such as career promotion, financial gain, or prestige.
- Regardless of study design, a financial conflict of interest is often associated with a more positive framing of study results in a way that favors the sponsor of the research.

Selecting children for the basketball team and an illustration of selection bias

Every year, between January 1 and December 31, a school basketball coach selects 100 children from each age category to enter the school's basketball team. To be fair and give every child a chance, the coach randomly selects children for the tryouts. Interestingly, in the age groups 6 through 12, most of the initially randomly selected children who finally made the team (12 players) were born in the first quarter of each year (January through March). They were the oldest and thus more likely to be the tallest in each age category.

The next year the school was competing in a basketball tournament with a neighboring school. To be fair, two children from each age group were selected at random for the team at each school. School 1 selected at random only children who were born between January and March, while school 2 selected those born throughout the year. School 1's process is an example of selection bias.

Selected readings

Akl EA, Hakoum M, Khamis A, Khabsa J, Vassar M, Guyatt G. A framework is proposed for defining, categorizing, and assessing conflicts of interest in health research. *J Clin Epidemiol.* 2022 Jun 11:S0895-4356(22)00147-0.

Higgins JPT, Savović J, Page MJ, Elbers RG, Sterne JAC. Chapter 8: Assessing risk of bias in a randomized trial. In: Higgins JPT, Thomas J, Chandler J, Cumpston M, Li T, Page MJ, Welch VA, eds. *Cochrane Handbook for Systematic Reviews of Interventions*, version 6.3 (updated February 2022). Cochrane, 2022. Available from www.training.cochrane.org/handbook.

Sackett DL. Bias in analytic research. *J Chronic Dis.* 1979;32(1–2):51–63.

Schulz KF. Assessing allocation concealment and blinding in randomised controlled trials: why bother? *Evidence-Based Nursing.* 2001;4:4–6.

Schulz KF, Chalmers I, Hayes RJ, Altman DG. Empirical evidence of bias. Dimensions of methodological quality associated with estimates of treatment effects in controlled trials. *JAMA.* 1995 Feb 1;273(5):408–412.

Sterne JAC, Hernán MA, McAleenan A, Reeves BC, Higgins JPT. Chapter 25: Assessing risk of bias in a non-randomized study. In: Higgins JPT, Thomas J, Chandler J, Cumpston M, Li T, Page MJ, Welch VA, eds. *Cochrane Handbook for Systematic Reviews of Interventions*, version 6.3 (updated February 2022). Cochrane, 2022. Available from www.training.cochrane.org/handbook.

14

Understanding and interpreting patient-reported outcomes

Patients, clinicians, and policymakers need to know the extent to which a treatment, new diagnostic test, or preventive intervention produces a net benefit in health. Determining what represents an improvement or deterioration in health status is an important aspect of modern health care and is directly related to a person-centered care approach—caring for a person with a disease rather than treating a disease in a patient. The determination of a person's health status varies depending on whom we ask—the patient or the doctor. In the past, clinicians used physiological, biological, or laboratory measures to evaluate clinical improvement or deterioration, assuming that such measures would provide an objective perspective of a person's health status. However, with the rise of chronic conditions and noncommunicable diseases and the abandonment of the paternalistic approach to decision making in favor of a more inclusive and person-centered framework, the focus of health *outcomes* has moved toward applying a patient's perspective to determine the value or impact that the provision of care has in their lives. This approach is now a priority for clinical research, health care agencies, and other stakeholders in the health system.

A patient's expectation or aspiration for achieving and maintaining optimal levels of oral health usually revolves around subjective aspects determined by their values and preferences. Relevant health outcomes important to a patient may include long-term tooth retention, satisfaction with their smile's esthetics, halitosis (bad breath), and the ability to speak, smell, chew, and swallow in a way that allows them to remain an integrated member of society across their life span. These health outcomes are sometimes described as quality-of-life-related domains that, when evaluated in the context of oral health, are referred to as *oral-health-related quality of life*. A *patient-* or *person-reported outcome* (PRO) is expressed as a *patient-* or *person-reported outcome measure* (PROM), which quantifies and tracks a person's health status or experience and is informed directly by that person, without interpretation of the response by a third party (e.g., clinician, proxy). PROMs aim to reflect a person's experience or perspective, which can be assessed only by the person themselves (Table 14.1).

The measurement of clinical attachment level, colony-forming units, degree of dysplasia in a potentially malignant lesion, or millimeters of face swelling or trismus requires calibrated instruments (e.g., periodontal probes, rulers with accuracy in millimeters, number of visible colonies present on an agar plate). Similarly, measuring PROs, such as the impact of oral diseases on a person's satisfaction with their smile, ability to chew or swallow, overall functioning, and level of confidence and well-being, requires the same level of precision and measurement rigor as other more clinically or laboratory-oriented measures. PROMs are indices, instruments, tools, or questionnaires developed to measure a PRO that provide critical information about a person's experience or perspective beyond clinical outcomes, such as biomarkers, morbidity measures, and

Statistics for Dental Clinicians, First Edition. Michael Glick, Alonso Carrasco-Labra, and Olivia Urquhart.
© 2024 John Wiley & Sons, Inc. Published 2024 by John Wiley & Sons, Inc.

Table 14.1   Type of patient-reported outcome measures, their advantages and limitations.

Type	Definition	Advantages	Limitations
1) Generic instruments	Cover the complete spectrum of health status (e.g., quality-of-life domains) and can be applied to a wide variety of populations.		
– Health profiles	Instruments designed to detect differential effects across a wide range of health status domains.	A single instrument can measure multiple aspects of health status. Designed to be used in a variety of populations, which allows for comparing treatment effects across different diseases or conditions.	As they cover a wide range of health status, they may fail to focus on a specific domain of interest, and therefore be unresponsive to the effect of a health care intervention of interest.
– Utility measures	Derived from economic and decision theory, they measure a person's preference and relate their health states to a continuum from full health (1.0) to death (0.0).	Allow for the conduct of cost-utility analysis (QALYs), with a wide variety of methods available (e.g., standard gamble, time trade-off). A single estimate represents the net impact of an intervention in health status.	Lack of sensitivity as to what aspect or domain of a person's health status is driving their response (i.e., single estimate reflecting both desirable and undesirable consequences). Potentially, unresponsive to the effect of a health care intervention.
2) Specific instruments	Focus on aspects of health status or problem that are specific to the area of primary interest, improving responsiveness and relevance. They can be specific to a disease (oral cancer), a symptom (pain), a function (speaking), or a population (children or older adults).	Their specificity increases the chance of the instrument to detect change overtime (i.e., responsiveness). Measure clinical features that clinicians routinely evaluate.	Narrow focus on a specific aspect of health status makes them not comprehensive to all aspects of a disease or condition. They cannot be used to compare the effect of an intervention across conditions.

QUALY = quality-adjusted life-years.

disease burden. Unfortunately, PROMs show a poor correlation with *performance-based outcomes*, physiological parameters, and *clinician-reported outcomes*. Yet patients and clinicians sometimes have no choice but to use only PROMs, for example, in conditions such as orofacial pain, acute and chronic pain, fatigue, depression, anxiety, and satisfaction with care. A PROM is designed to meet at least one of the following purposes to inform clinical practice or research:

1) Discriminate. These instruments should be used when there is a need to classify or distinguish individuals or groups of individuals according to a particular person's feature, at a single point in time (cross-sectional), in the absence of an external criterion or gold standard to validate the measure. An example is the use of a visual analog scale of pain to discriminate among patients with different pain intensity levels.

2) Predict. These instruments attempt to predict, classify, or identify people with a specific set of features or categories for which an external criterion or gold standard is available. This external criterion is then used to determine whether individuals have been correctly classified by the predictive instrument. These tools identify individuals who will or will not develop a particular condition or outcome in the future. As an external criterion is already available, a new instrument for predicting should offer additional advantages compared to that criterion. For example, the new instrument or questionnaire should be less invasive, cheaper, and easier to administer, with less burden for the clinician or the patient. An example of such an instrument is the use of a reliable and valid caries risk assessment tool providing information regarding the absolute risk of experiencing a caries lesion for a particular timeframe.

3) Evaluate. An instrument can be designed to measure the magnitude of change (e.g., large, moderate, small but important, trivial, no change at all) from baseline in an individual's trait or health status. In other words, such an instrument is sensitive to change over time (longitudinal), a property particularly relevant when using PROMs in clinical trials testing the effect of an intervention. An example of such an instrument is an oral-health-related quality-of-life instrument proven to be sensitive to change between times 1 and 2.

As PROMs are designed to meet a specific purpose and measure a particular *construct*, clinicians should be aware that not all of them are created equal. It is necessary to examine whether a PROM of interest is trustworthy to inform practice.

Identifying optimal patient-reported outcome measures

In the same way that we demand instruments measuring blood pressure, clinical attachment level, body temperature, and mouth opening to provide accurate results (e.g., appropriately calibrated, consistent results over time), PROMs also need to demonstrate that they are useful and meet the required measurement properties. Researchers developing PROMs need to provide evidence of the following measurement properties:

Validity

A valid PROM is an instrument (e.g., a health questionnaire) that measures the underlying construct as intended. For example, a sphygmomanometer measures the construct of blood pressure, which corresponds to the force of circulating blood against the walls of the arteries. Although the word "construct" might be unfamiliar to clinicians, they might be familiar with the meaning as they identify constructs associated with their patients' conditions. The presence of disease, the severity of signs and symptoms, and the excess or deficit of a biological variable are all examples of constructs. Researchers developing PROMs increase their *validity* by including questions developed in consultation with patients who have experienced the condition of interest or their caregivers or parents who are aware of the disease and its impact on their lives (formally called *face validity*). PROM developers can also consult with clinicians who have expertise in managing the disease who can determine whether the instrument appropriately covers all the aspects of the construct (*content validity*). *Construct validity*, generated by a process emanating from multiple research studies intended to ascertain that a PROM score or a result is valid, is a vital concept as it allows drawing accurate conclusions about the construct of interest or health status.

Reliability

In the world of health measurements, *reliability* refers to the extent to which a PROM is able to provide consistent results, free of measurement errors. Reliability is measured as a ratio of the variability in scores in a PROM between persons (between-person variability) to the total variability (i.e., between and within-person variability). A perfect instrument with no *random error* will have a reliability estimate equal to 1.0. As the magnitude of total variability increases (denominator) compared to the between-person variability (numerator), the reliability approaches zero. Typically, researchers provide two measures of reliability: (1) *Cohen's kappa (κ)*, which measures agreement between two or more observers (*inter-rater reliability*) or between two or more time points (*intra-rater reliability*), taking into account the possibility of the agreement occurring by chance (for *categorical variables*) (Appendix 1, Equation 14.1), and (2) the intraclass correlation coefficient (for *continuous variables*).

A hypothetical scenario—Cohen's kappa (k)

In a first scenario, two clinicians evaluated the presence or absence of noncavitated caries lesions with dental radiographs. Their record of agreement was calculated to be 80%. In a second scenario, two independent clinicians who had no idea how to determine the presence of noncavitated caries lesions reviewed 100 dental radiographs. As they had no previous training, they could only guess at the presence or absence of noncavitated caries lesions. Thus, we can expect that they would agree half of the time just by chance (Table 14.2), so that of the 100% of total possible agreement, 50% is simply due to chance. Although the clinicians in the first scenario calculated an 80% agreement (raw agreement), their clinical skills account for just 30% of that agreement. The kappa statistic corresponds to the quotient of the difference in the observed (raw) agreement (80%) and the expected agreement (agreement by chance alone; 50%) (Figure 14.1). In the example above, the raw agreement between the two clinicians was 80%. After correcting for agreement by chance—their diagnosis of a noncavitated caries lesion just by guessing—the corrected measure of agreement dropped to 60% (Appendix 1, Equation 14.1).

Consider this example to better understand the many aspects of reliability. To determine where to install a bookshelf, the space needs to be measured accurately. A retractable tape measure showing meters and subdivided is used. The tape measure should adhere to the established definition (*gold standard*) of a meter (the length of the path traveled by light in a vacuum during a specific amount of time—1/299,792,458 in a second (m/s), where the second is defined as "the time

Table 14.2 Representation of agreement between two clinicians who are not trained to diagnose the presence of noncavitated caries lesions and they are just guessing whether a lesion is present or absent (agreement just by chance alone).

		Clinician 1		
		Correct	Incorrect	
Clinician 2	Correct	**25**	25	50
	Incorrect	25	**25**	50
		50	50	100

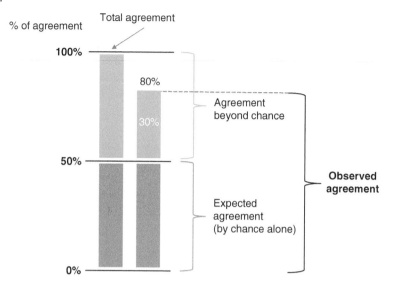

Figure 14.1 Proportion of total agreement (100%) in relation to expected agreement (50%) and agreement beyond chance (30%) when calculating Kappa statistic (chance-corrected agreement). Chance-corrected agreement for an observed agreement of 80% (raw agreement).

duration of 9,192,631,770 periods of the radiation corresponding to the transition between the two hyperfine levels of the fundamental unperturbed ground-state of the caesium-133 atom").[1] If manufacturers followed the standard above, the meter in the tape measure would match the original meter (the used measure, meter, is *valid* as it measures what it is intended to measure).

The width and height of the available space are measured. The same person conducts three consecutive separate measurements to ensure there is no mistake (intra-rater reliability). A second person completes the same process to ascertain if the measure of the two persons matches (inter-rater reliability). To improve the reliability of all the measures done to this point, the first person conducts an additional measurement of the available space (*test-retest reliability*). Although every measure presented above represents a possibility for incurring measurement errors, there is a breadth of indirect evidence suggesting that using this particular retractable tape measure is a reliable way to determine the size of the available space.

These examples are oversimplifications. Two crucial assumptions about the above concepts are, for the most part, hardly ever applicable to PROMs: (1) we do have a gold standard for the length of a meter, while for a PROM we do not; and (2) the example assumes that the wall never changed, which is rarely the case when measuring a person's health status.

One last element of reliability corresponds to *internal consistency*, which determines the extent to which the items or questions in an instrument relate to each other, reflecting the same construct. Cronbach's alpha is one of the most frequently used estimates to determine internal consistency.

Responsiveness

Investigators developing a PROM may provide evidence of reliability and validity, which can help users to trust that their measure of patients' health status is appropriate (e.g., PROMs with

---

1 The International System of Units. International Bureau of Weights and Measures. 9th edition, France.

discriminative or predictive purposes). Clinicians using PROMs in their practice and researchers conducting clinical trials compare the health status of a patient or study participant before and after the application of a treatment or preventive intervention. By doing so, they are trying to detect whether the person receiving the intervention experienced a change (i.e., improvement or deterioration) in their health status as measured by the PROM. Responsiveness refers to the ability of a PROM to detect change over time in the construct of interest. To study this property, researchers conduct a longitudinal study recruiting participants known to change over time on the construct of interest. Then, they assess the detection ability of the instrument to that change by, for example, correlating the change in the PROM with the change in other variables related to the construct of interest.

A few additional notes

- PROMs offer measures of what matters to people, patients, and society overall. They have been presented as the cornerstone of people-oriented health care frameworks like value-based care. The use of these outcomes, however, comes with challenges. Besides the need to utilize reliable, valid, and responsive measures, PROMs should enable interpretation of the magnitude of the impact (i.e., effect) of an intervention. The magnitude of an effect reflects the extent to which the observed results correspond to a trivial, small but important, moderate, or large effect.
- The need to distinguish magnitudes of effect, for example, being able to differentiate trivial or unimportant from effects that are small yet important to patients, led to the development of *minimal important difference* (MID) (Chapter 20). MID corresponds to the smallest within-person change in the score of an outcome (beneficial or harmful) that people perceive as important.

How much tooth whitening is right: An application of patient-reported outcome measures to tooth whitening techniques

Oral health encompasses a broad and diverse set of domains that go beyond the absence of disease. The ability to smile with confidence is part of these domains.[2] Tooth whitening is one of the most commonly used interventions in dentistry, as having white teeth is highly regarded in many areas of the world, particularly North America. With a large demand for whitening services, investigators have conducted extensive research to determine its benefits and harms and the size of those effects. A series of whitening enhancement techniques are available, including ozone, LED lights, lasers, and multiple combinations of doses and vehicles of administration. How can we determine the extent to which any of these enhancements and dose modifications truly affects the size of the effect? Is it worth implementing these enhancement techniques? Who should determine this, and based on what outcomes? One option is to use predetermined tooth shade scales that calibrated clinicians apply before and after the whitening application (clinician-rated). To objectively measure whitening changes, others use chroma meter devices (machine-rated). A third option would be to ask the patient, "Compared to your previous

---

2 Glick M, Williams DM, Kleinman DV, Vujicic M, Watt RG, Weyant RJ. A new definition for oral health developed by the FDI World Dental Federation opens the door to a universal definition of oral health. *J Am Dent Assoc.* 2016 Dec;147(12):915–917.

perception of tooth color, how satisfied are you with the color after the whitening agent was applied?" (patient-reported). Each of these measures has pros and cons and intrinsic meaning and importance. For example, would we consider a whitening agent showing significant changes in a clinician- and machine-rated outcome measures but no difference in a patient-reported outcome measure effective? "The client is always right" is a common expression in businesses where there is no objective measure to establish the quality or value of a product and the client determines the perceived value. With the emergence of a person-centered approach to care, future research, including tooth whitening studies, should move toward a more person-reported type of outcome approach. In health care, the client may not always be right; however, the days when researchers reported their outcome measures disregarding the patient perspective are in the past.

Selected readings

Calvert M, Kyte D, Price G, Valderas JM, Hjollund NH. Maximising the impact of patient reported outcome assessment for patients and society. *BMJ.* 2019;364:k5267.

Carrasco-Labra A, Devji T, Qasim A, et al. Minimal important difference estimates for patient-reported outcomes: a systematic survey. *J Clin Epidemiol.* 2021 May;133:61–71.

Cella D, Hahn EA, Jensen SE, Butt Z, Nowinski CJ, Rothrock N, Lohr KN. *Patient-Reported Outcomes in Performance Measurement.* RTI Press; 2015 Sep. Types of Patient-Reported Outcomes. https://www.ncbi.nlm.nih.gov/books/NBK424381/.

Hancock SL, Ryan OF, Marion V, et al. Feedback of patient-reported outcomes to healthcare professionals for comparing health service performance: a scoping review. *BMJ Open.* 2020;10:e038190.

Johnston BC, Patrick DL, Devji T, et al. Patient-reported outcomes. In: Higgins JPT, Thomas J, Chandler J, Cumpston M, Li T, Page MJ, Welch VA, eds. *Cochrane Handbook for Systematic Reviews of Interventions*, version 6.3 (updated February 2022). Cochrane; 2022. www.training.cochrane.org/handbook.

Kluzek S, Dean B, Wartolowska KA. Patient-reported outcome measures (PROMs) as proof of treatment efficacy. *BMJ Evidence-Based Medicine.* 2022;27:153–155.

McGinn T, Wyer PC, Newman TB, Keitz S, Leipzig R, For GG; Evidence-Based Medicine Teaching Tips Working Group. Tips for learners of evidence-based medicine: 3. Measures of observer variability (kappa statistic). *CMAJ.* 2004 Nov 23;171(11):1369–1373.

15

Understanding and interpreting a cross-sectional study

Observational studies can be *analytical or descriptive. Case-control studies* (Chapter 16) and *cohort studies* (Chapter 17) are classic examples of research utilizing analytical designs to establish an *association* between an *exposure* and an *outcome*. To establish such an association, analytical studies require a *control group* that serves as a reference to estimate the magnitude of the relationship. Descriptive studies, on the other hand, depict a phenomenon, such as the *frequency* of a disease or condition in a *population*.

Cross-sectional studies can be analytical, providing information of a potential association between an exposure and an outcome, but also descriptive, providing information about disease *prevalence*, or the frequency, of a characteristic in a population. However, cross-sectional research, as opposed to case-control and cohort studies, collects data at a single point in time, providing a snapshot of variables of interest. Both exposures and outcomes are measured simultaneously, disregarding their temporality (i.e., whether the exposure occurred before the outcome or whether the outcome occurred before the exposure). The data-collection process can be designed de novo (anew) or can take advantage of existing data records. When conducting de novo cross-sectional studies, such as surveys, investigators can utilize valid and reliable instruments and questionnaires to ascertain the exposures and outcomes of interest, have the opportunity to ensure that those who collect data are calibrated, and apply rigorous methods to determine participants' eligibility. Many of these advantages are unavailable when conducting a cross-sectional study using existing health records (Figure 15.1).

Bias in cross-sectional studies

Bias or *systematic error* (Chapter 13) in a cross-sectional study has the potential to produce misleading results that fail to reflect the true prevalence of the population of interest or spurious associations between exposures and outcomes. Biases can be classified into two main categories—selection bias and information bias.

Selection bias is a family of biases that can affect the *external validity* of a cross-sectional study; it arises from the drawing of a *sample* that is not representative of the population of interest. Several scenarios can introduce selection bias. *Sampling bias* ensues when some individuals from the population of interest are more likely than other individuals to be enrolled in the study (nonrandom selection). *Nonresponse bias* occurs when important differences exist between responders and nonresponders to a survey or questionnaire. *Prevalence-incidence or Neyman bias* arises when the sampling process facilitates the inclusion of a disproportionally high percentage of individuals with the outcome of interest or cases with long disease duration over other individuals with a more severe progression and shorter duration, which would prevent or minimize their chances of being sampled.

Statistics for Dental Clinicians, First Edition. Michael Glick, Alonso Carrasco-Labra, and Olivia Urquhart.
© 2024 John Wiley & Sons, Inc. Published 2024 by John Wiley & Sons, Inc.

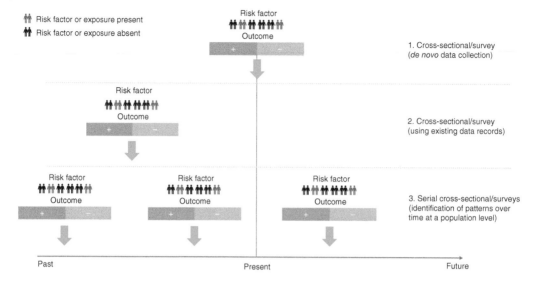

Figure 15.1 Three types of cross-sectional study designs according to data collection method over time. Blue horizontal arrows represent a timeline from past to future. The vertical blue line represents the present time. Red figures depict individuals exposed to a risk factor of interest while black figures depict individuals unexposed to a risk factor of interest. A green box with a + sign reflects the presence of an outcome of interest while a yellow box with a - sign reflects the absence of an outcome of interest. Risk factors and outcomes are measured simultaneously in this type of design. The green arrow pointing down illustrates data at a single point in time.

Information bias is a group of biases that can affect the validity of a cross-sectional study when investigators fail to appropriately measure and interpret the data. *Observer bias* ensues when investigators are aware of the disease status or outcome of interest and ask leading questions so that participants' responses confirm the investigators' hypothesis. *Recall bias* arises when study participants' disease status affects their likelihood of reporting an exposure. For example, a study participant with lung cancer may be more likely than one without lung cancer to recall having used tobacco in their youth; or a study participant suffering from a particular mental disorder may not recall an exposure. *Detection bias* occurs when the ascertainment or measurement of the disease or outcome of interest is systematically different between exposed and unexposed groups.

Response rate and avoiding nonresponse

The response rate is an important measure when interpreting results from a survey. Users of evidence from cross-sectional studies should examine the magnitude of response rates and evaluate to what extent there are reasons to suspect that those responding to the survey were systematically different from those who were identified yet did not respond. For example, if a response rate is only 5%, do the other 95% of individuals invited to respond differ in some important way from the responders? It is recognized that individual characteristics, such as age, gender, education level, cultural background, or features of the study, including sampling methods and length or complexity of the data-collection instrument or questionnaire, are factors influencing a response rate. Among the strategies that investigators can use to limit the impact of nonresponse issues are designing simple, short, and intuitive questionnaires with an academic pitch rather than a commercial angle, giving eligible individuals notice that a survey is arriving soon, issuing incentives, and following up with nonresponders.

Analysis of cross-sectional studies

Analyses of cross-sectional studies are conducted according to the primary objective of the study (e.g., descriptive, analytical) and include descriptive analyses, standard statistical hypothesis testing (see Chapter 5), and *regression* modeling (Chapter 11). *Confounding* (Chapter 12) is another issue to consider in analytical cross-sectional studies; investigators can control for *confounders* using a combination of strategies, including specific study design considerations (e.g., specification or restriction, stratification, matching) and statistical analysis considerations (e.g., multivariable regression analysis) (Chapter 11).

In descriptive cross-sectional studies, investigators focus on frequency measures. The prevalence, one of the most important findings in a cross-sectional study, is a measure of the number of cases of, for example, a disease in a population of interest at a specific time point as a proportion of the total number of individuals in the population. Prevalence does not exclude individuals who were diagnosed with a disease and then recovered within the timeframe of interest but does not include new cases identified outside of the period examined. This timeframe may be a single point in time (e.g., the prevalence of COVID-19 in the United States on March 19, 2020), called *point prevalence*, or the number of cases over a time interval, called *period prevalence* (e.g., the prevalence of COVID-19 in the United States during 2020). Table 15.1. includes cross-tabulated data for a hypothetical cross-sectional study assessing the prevalence of a disease among exposed and unexposed individuals. From the table, three estimates, descriptive in nature, can be calculated: prevalence for the whole population (10%) (Appendix 1, Equation 15.1), prevalence among those exposed (20%) (Appendix 1, Equation 15.2), and prevalence among the unexposed (6.7%) (Appendix 1, Equation 15.3). In addition, two additional estimates allow the exploration of associations between exposure and outcomes or the presence of disease. The *prevalence odds ratio* (POR) calculated the same way as any *odds ratio* (Chapter 2), compares the odds of having the disease between exposed and unexposed groups. A POR of 3.5 (Appendix 1, Equation 15.4) means that the odds of having the disease among exposed people is 3.5 times as high as the odds of having the disease among unexposed people (Chapter 2). Another measure of association specific to analytical cross-sectional studies is the *prevalence ratio* (PR). The PR is analogous to a risk ratio (Chapter 2) and is calculated in a similar way. In our hypothetical example (Table 15.1), the PR = 3.0 (Appendix 1, Equation 15.5), which means that the proportion of people with the disease is 3.0 times as high among the exposed compared to the unexposed.

Table 15.1 Estimates in descriptive and analytical cross-sectional studies.

	Condition present	Condition absent	Total
Exposure present (exposed)	100[a]	400[b]	500
Exposure absent (unexposed)	100[c]	1,400[d]	1,500
Total	200	1,800	2,000

[a] Exposed individuals with the condition.
[b] Exposed individuals without the condition.
[c] Unexposed individuals with the condition.
[d] Unexposed individuals without the condition.

Advantages and limitations of a cross-sectional study

First, cross-sectional studies are less expensive to conduct compared to those that are longitudinal in nature, such as cohort studies (Chapter 17) and randomized controlled trials (Chapter 18). Second, a major advantage of cross-sectional studies is that there is no time between the measurement of the exposure or risk factor and the outcome, which means that loss to follow-up is a non-issue. Third, cross-sectional studies are helpful in determining diagnostic test accuracy of an index test against a reference test (a gold standard) for individuals suspected to have a disease or seemingly healthy individuals (Chapter 9). Fourth, this study design is an efficient way to ascertain an association between exposures, or personal characteristics, and an outcome where the exposure and the outcome occur within a very short timeframe (e.g., within a few hours or a day). However, since only prevalence as opposed to incidence data (a measure of the number of new cases that develop over a particular period) can be collected, any statement of cause and effect, prognosis, or disease progression should be considered with a high degree of skepticism. The lack of temporal sequence between exposure and outcome in analytical cross-sectional studies can misguide users by making them assume that one factor is causing an outcome when the relationship could be the opposite.

A few additional notes

- Cross-sectional studies are used as hypothesis-generating tools to evaluate disease etiology.
- The most common type of cross-sectional study is that which measures the prevalence of diseases or the frequency of a particular health status in the population, for example, a national survey. The availability of prevalence information can facilitate planning for administrators and public health personnel to learn about the health status of the people they serve and determine resource allocation for preventive and therapeutic efforts. Additionally, they provide preliminary evidence to explore etiological (risk) factors for a population of interest. Further, the results of prevalence studies help clinicians to assess the likelihood or pretest probability of disease, which is used to determine positive and negative predictive values for a diagnostic test (Chapter 9) but also specific conditions in the population they serve. For example, oral leukoplakia is a white-plaque lesion in the oral mucosa of unknown origin and is worrisome in adults 50 or older. Among oral white lesions, leukoplakia has a prevalence ranging between 1.5% and 2.6%. Thus, out of 100 white lesions a clinician observes among adults 50 years or older, roughly only two or three of those will be oral leukoplakias. However, 97 or 98 will have a different diagnosis. In contrast, a differential diagnosis of a white-plaque-like lesion with a similar clinical appearance but this time in a newborn should include at the top of the list of differential diagnoses the possibility of a superficial candida infection, which has a prevalence ranging between 5% and 10%. The higher the prevalence of a disease in a population, the higher that diagnosis will rank in the diagnostic workup. A special type of study of disease prevalence is a national health survey, which documents the frequency of health-related behaviors, risk factors, disease burdens, and health care needs. Regional- or country-level surveys provide data regarding a population's health status to assist administrators, payers, and policy makers in informing an agenda conducive to addressing the issues that the survey identified. When applied repeatedly over time (time trend approach) and as part of public health planning, national surveys allow for epidemiological surveillance and monitoring of possible changes in population health parameters. The data collected in these surveys are often available through public databases that researchers can access to conduct hypothesis-generating secondary analyses. The fundamental requirement for

any national cross-sectional study is obtaining a sample representative of the underlying population of interest. Country-level cross-sectional studies are often conducted as *serial surveys*, administered with a certain periodicity, such as every five years. This design not only provides a snapshot of the population's status at the time point of data collection but also highlights changes in patterns over time when comparing one period with another or several consecutive periods (Figure 15.1). Although national serial surveys over 20 or 30 years allow investigators to conduct longitudinal analyses comparing different periods, they are different from cohort studies (Chapter 17). Every period in a serial survey requires a new representative sample from the population of interest. This means that only group-level or sample-level, not individual-level, findings are valid as long as every serial sample is representative of the population. In contrast, in a cohort study, the same individuals initially enrolled are followed prospectively, which allows researchers to determine the association between exposures or risk factors and outcomes or diseases at an individual level.

- Cross-sectional studies can also provide preliminary evidence of an association between exposure and outcome or the presence of disease. In this type of design, investigators measure the presence or absence of risk factors (i.e., exposure) and the presence of a disease (i.e., outcome) simultaneously for every enrolled participant—an example of an *etiological study*. The cases of the disease or participants in the study presenting the outcome are "prevalent cases." This means that the investigators are aware of every participant having and not having the exposure and outcome of interest; however, they do not know the sequence of events (i.e., exposure to disease) or the duration between exposure and outcome. This issue makes any identified exposure/outcome association hypothetical. The inability to determine the directionality of events makes cross-sectional studies prone to *temporality bias*, also known as *reverse causality* or *antecedent-consequent bias* (see the pullout box for an example).

- Identifying individuals with a feature of interest who will be part of the study sample is an essential step when conducting cross-sectional studies. When participants are identified correctly, the study results can be generalized from the study sample back to the population of interest. Researchers conducting cross-sectional studies use two major types of sampling methods. The first type corresponds to a *probabilistic sampling* approach, in which the investigators identify participants using probability theory. The key feature of this type of sampling is that any individual in the population of interest has the same probability of being selected for the study. Then, individuals are randomly chosen. This is referred to as *simple random sampling*. A second approach allows investigators to identify eligible individuals by selecting them using a specific unit of sampling. For example, out of 1,000 eligible individuals numbered from 1 to 1,000, researchers can determine to systematically select one participant for every 20 individuals. This method is referred to as *systematic sampling*. A third approach is known as *stratified sampling*. This technique is used when a specific variable of interest, such as gender, is specific to nonoverlapping groups or strata. In other words, investigators divide the entire population of interest into two groups, such as males and females, and draw a random sample within each group (stratum). A fourth approach is *cluster sampling*, used when eligible individuals for a study naturally cluster in discrete geographic or organizational units. These clusters can be municipalities, hospitals, schools, or classes and become the unit of sampling from which investigators can draw a simple random sample. Cross-sectional studies with optimal probabilistic sampling often include a combination of the approaches presented above in what is called *multistage sampling*. For example, the Centers for Disease Control and Prevention, in conducting the National Health and Nutrition Examination Survey (NHANES), identifies counties as single sampling units in the first stage. Then the counties are further divided into smaller units limited by city blocks and sampled according to their size. In the third stage, the households in each sample unit are identified, and a random sample of the households is taken. In the last stage, individuals within the randomly selected households are identified; again, a random sample of individuals within each household is taken, and on average two persons are included per eligible household. In addition, the NHANES survey oversamples subgroups of the population (e.g., adolescents, minorities) to increase the trustworthiness and *precision* of health status estimates for these groups. The second group of methods includes the *nonprobabilistic sampling* approaches, which use not probabilities but convenience or subjective criteria to identify the study sample. These approaches are particularly helpful when a complete identification of the entire population of interest is impossible or very challenging. The most common nonprobabilistic approach is the selection of individuals based on their availability or willingness to participate in the study. This approach is often used in clinical or health care units that recruit participants who are primarily seeking care and are conveniently invited to participate in the study; this is called *convenience sampling*. A second nonprobabilistic approach, called *purposive sampling*, includes the identification of participants based on the study purpose or a set of subjective characteristics used as eligibility criteria. In a third approach, known as *snowball sampling*, where enrolled individuals invite their peers satisfying the eligibility criteria. This method is particularly helpful when studying sensitive topics or addressing close-knit communities that are difficult to penetrate for investigators but easily accessible to members of the community.

The chicken or egg dilemma: antecedent-consequent bias or reverse causality in cross-sectional studies (Figure 15.2).

Consider a hypothetical cross-sectional study conducted in a large dental service organization. To determine if there is an association between chronic respiratory disease and the fabrication and adjustment of dentures, 100 clinicians are identified as those who fabricate and adjust dentures (exposed group) and 100 clinicians are identified as those who do not fabricate and adjust dentures (unexposed group). Data collected at time 1 suggest that five times as many clinicians who fabricate and adjust dentures have a chronic respiratory disease as compared with clinicians who do not fabricate and adjust dentures (prevalence ratio time 1 = 5.0).

Suppose data are collected a second time—time 2. Now the results suggest a greater prevalence of chronic respiratory disease among clinicians who do not fabricate and adjust dentures (unexposed group) instead of among clinicians who fabricate and adjust dentures (exposed group) (prevalence ratio time 2 = 0.7).

This change in prevalence ratio is not attributable to not fabricating and adjusting dentures suddenly becoming a hazardous exposure. It is the result of 15 clinicians who did fabricate and adjust dentures initially no longer doing so, possibly because of their chronic respiratory symptoms. Thus, at time 2, for a number of clinicians with chronic respiratory disease (n = 15) who no longer fabricate and adjust dentures, the effect or consequence of their symptoms, not their hypothesized cause (fabricating and adjusting dentures), has moved them from the exposed group to the nonexposed group.

By design, cross-sectional studies are irreversibly affected by reverse causation, also known as antecedent-consequent bias (chicken or egg dilemma), because the temporal sequence between exposure and outcome cannot be determined. Since both exposure and outcome are measured simultaneously, cross-sectionally, it cannot be defined whether the exposure preceded or resulted from the occurrence of the outcome or disease. This is not the case in cohort studies (Chapter 17) or randomized controlled trials (Chapter 18), which provide more robust evidence for causal inference, with clear ascertainment that the exposure or experimental intervention occurred before the outcome of interest was observed.

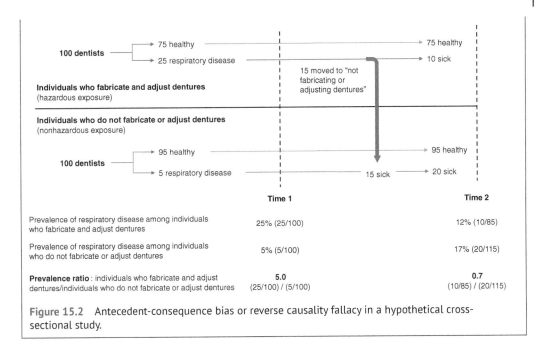

Figure 15.2 Antecedent-consequence bias or reverse causality fallacy in a hypothetical cross-sectional study.

Selected readings

Sedgwick P. Bias in observational study designs: cross sectional studies. *BMJ.* 2015 Mar 6;350:h1286.

Sedgwick P. Multistage sampling. *BMJ.* 2015 Jul 31;351:h4155.

Wang X, Cheng Z. Cross-sectional studies: strengths, weaknesses, and recommendations. *Chest.* 2020 Jul;158(1S):S65–S71.

16

Understanding and interpreting a case-control study

In a *case-control study*, two groups of individuals—with (*cases*) and without (*controls*) the *outcome* or disease/condition of interest (often an infrequent disease)—are identified to determine the *proportion* of individuals in each group who have certain characteristics or have been exposed to a *risk factor* in the past. For simplicity, from here on in, the word "outcome" will encompass individuals with a disease or condition. Case-control studies are retrospective in nature—the measurement of the *exposure* occurs after the outcome is observed, which is the opposite of the expected exposure → outcome temporal sequence (Figure 16.1). Along with *cohort studies* (Chapter 17) and analytical *cross-sectional studies* (Chapter 15), well-conducted and comprehensively reported case-control studies can provide valuable evidence of an *association* between exposure and an outcome of interest.

Selection of the *study population*

Out of the general population, investigators determine eligibility criteria and define a narrower study population, composed of individuals with (cases) and without (controls) the outcome of interest (black figures in Figure 16.2). A sample of that study population is drawn and enrolled in the study without awareness of their exposure status. If the investigators select cases or controls for the study depending on their exposure, the case-control study is at high risk of *bias* (Figure 16.2).

Identifying cases

The selection of cases in a case-control study should ideally comply with the sampling principles applied to other epidemiological study designs—the sample of cases should be representative of the broad population of cases that exist at a particular time and would benefit from the study results. There are two types of cases. *Prevalent cases* are those individuals who already experienced the outcome of interest at some point in the past within the observation period (Figure 16.1). When using prevalent cases, investigators should report the study results using *prevalence odds ratios* (Chapter 15). *Incident cases* are those individuals who recently developed the outcome of interest within the observation period (Figure 16.1). Incident cases are preferred to prevalent cases, especially when the purpose of the study is to determine the role that risk factors play in the outcome of interest. The population of cases can be defined in a number of ways, depending on their particular demographic characteristics, disease features and severity, geographical location, and health care coverage. When the *frequency* of the outcome of interest is very low, a suitable scenario

Statistics for Dental Clinicians, First Edition. Michael Glick, Alonso Carrasco-Labra, and Olivia Urquhart.
© 2024 John Wiley & Sons, Inc. Published 2024 by John Wiley & Sons, Inc.

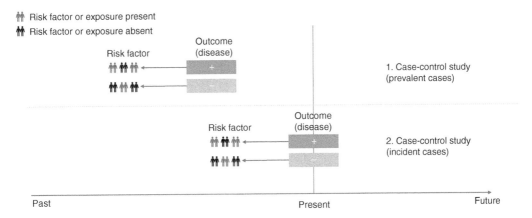

Figure 16.1 Case-control study design using prevalent and incident cases. Blue horizontal arrows represent a timeline from past to future. The vertical blue line represents the present time. Red figures depict individuals exposed to a risk factor of interest while black figures depict individuals unexposed to a risk factor of interest. A green box with a + sign reflects the presence of an outcome of interest while a yellow box with a - sign reflects the absence of an outcome of interest. Risk factors and outcomes are measured simultaneously in this type of design. The blue arrows pointing to the past (to the left) illustrate the retrospective aspect of the study design, i.e., the assessment of the association of interest starts from cases and controls and goes back in time to determine the presence or absence of potential risk factors.

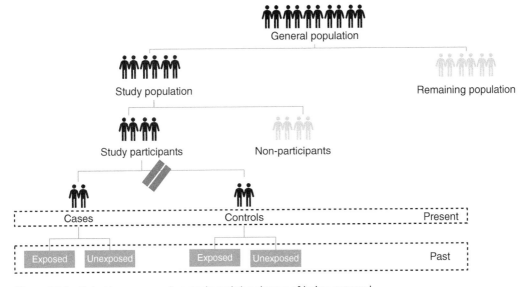

Figure 16.2 Selecting cases and controls and the chance of being exposed.

for a case-control study, investigators take advantage of discipline-specific registries or highly specialized clinical and research centers or hospitals managing a large volume of referrals to identify cases. The downside of this apparent convenience is that the cases' representativeness of the population of interest is questionable. A solution to this issue is to include cases from several hospitals or research centers across a region or country. The diagnostic means to identify a case as such are critical and should be based on objective diagnostic criteria supported by optimal levels of test *sensitivity* and *specificity*. Specificity is of special interest because the unexpected inclusion in the case group of a participant with a false positive result would dilute any potential association.

Identifying controls

Selecting controls is one of the most challenging steps in a case-control study. The primary goal here is to identify outcome- or disease-free individuals from a population such that if the outcome occurs, they would be eligible as cases (Figure 16.2). There are three main sampling methods used to identify controls:

- Institution- (e.g., hospital, clinic, research center) or registry-based controls. Because of convenience, investigators often identify controls from the same hospital, clinic, or registry where they identified cases. The main problem with this approach is that if the exposure of interest results in individuals developing a medical issue that subsequently makes them seek health care, the frequency of the exposure among controls will be misleadingly high. This spuriously high frequency of exposure among controls can bias the association, obliterating it or even reversing its direction. This type of bias is called *hospital patient bias* or *Berkson's bias*.
- Population-based sampling using databases. Extensive population-level clinical and administrative databases have facilitated the conduct of population-based case-control studies. Cases identified through extensive registries are more representative of the population of cases of interest compared to those sampled from a single hospital or clinic. Consequently, the identified controls tend to be more representative of the population without the outcome of interest. The more comprehensive, centralized, and stable a database, the higher the *generalizability* of the case-control study.
- Combination of approaches. The difficulty in identifying and selecting controls for an unbiased comparison of the frequency of exposure with the cases has guided some investigators to obtain more than one sample of controls. If the measure of association (i.e., odds ratio) is similar when different control groups are compared to the cases, the validity of the study findings increases.

Retrospective assessment of the exposure

Retrospective assessment of the exposure is one of the main challenges in a case-control study. In many studies, information provided by the participants is the single source for determining if an exposure occurred. The further back in time the exposure occurred, the more prone the study is to be affected by *misclassification bias*. Relying only on participants' memory is a major limitation of case-control studies. It is possible that the cases, as they have experienced the outcome of interest, may be more prone to remember and report being exposed to a risk factor when in reality they were unexposed (*differential misclassification bias* of the exposure). This issue is a classic type of misclassification in case-control studies called *recall bias*. In other situations, cases and controls may both be prone to inaccurately recollecting an exposure in their past, like their exercise habits 10 years ago (*nondifferential misclassification bias*). To minimize misclassification bias and to increase the fidelity of the reported status on the exposure in cases and controls, investigators use a series of strategies and tools. They can blind participants to the primary measure of the exposure or risk factor by asking them about the exposure of interest among multiple "dummy" and unrelated exposures. In addition, if the outcome of interest is not evidently observable, the investigators collecting information about the exposure status can also be blinded to whether the participant is a case or a control. During the data-collection process, investigators can take advantage of standardized questionnaires including pictures or other diagrams to represent the exposures of interest. The application of the same questionnaires to both cases and controls reduces the possibility of

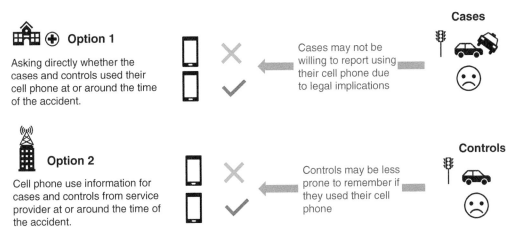

Figure 16.3 Hypothetical study to determine the association between texting while driving (exposure) and the occurrence of motor vehicle accidents (outcome), and options to measure the exposure between cases and controls.

misclassification bias resulting in a spurious association. Another strategy to minimize misclassification bias is the utilization of different sources of information, which can then be cross-verified. For example, Figure 16.3 shows a hypothetical case-control study conducted with the purpose of determining whether there is an association between texting while driving (exposure) and motor vehicle accidents (outcome). Investigators may ask cases and controls directly whether they used their phones at or around the time of the accident, but this method has several limitations. For example, the cases may not be willing to report phone usage due to potential legal implications. In addition, investigators may be missing the more severe cases who were referred immediately for emergency surgery as their health status prevented them from being interviewed to ascertain their phone usage (exposure). And controls might have difficulty remembering whether they were on their cell phones at a particular time on a typical day. The second option for the investigators would be to obtain information regarding cell phone usage at or around the time of the accident directly from service providers. This data-collection strategy will increase the fidelity of the data among cases and controls and solve the methodological issues presented above with option 1. Data cross-referencing using existing records is a valuable strategy to increase the fidelity of the measurement of the exposure. Clinical and pharmacy records, radiographs, laboratory measurements, and other types of clinical registries can serve as sources for cross-referencing data. One limitation of these sources is that in most cases they were not intended for use in research or to measure the exposure in the manner that the study requires.

As with any other observational study design, case-control studies require controlling for confounding variables (Chapter 12). This can be done at the design phase by implementing *specification (restriction)* or *matching*. To adjust for confounders at the analysis level, stratification and *logistic regression* modeling can also be used.

Once data are collected to ascertain exposure status, investigators determine the *proportion* of cases and controls exposed to one or more risk factors of interest. Since the number of cases in the study is determined arbitrarily by the investigator (informed by a formal sample size calculation), it is impossible to determine a measure of incidence for the outcome of interest. To make sense of the data, an *odds ratio*, including the *odds* of being exposed to a risk factor in the cases, is compared to the odds of being exposed among subjects in the control group (Chapter 2). An odds ratio = 1 means that the odds of exposure are the same among cases and controls. An odds ratio > 1 means that those with the disease are more likely to be exposed than those without the disease. An odds ratio < 1 means that those with the disease are less likely to be exposed than those without the disease. For example, a hypothetical case-control study assessed the association between exposure to dental radiographs and having head and neck cancer. The cases were selected from a large state of Pennsylvania database and were all confirmed with biopsy. The controls were identified from similar geographical locations in Pennsylvania and were matched according to age and sex; none had a previous or current diagnosis of head and neck cancer. The calculated odds ratio for this association was 1.17, meaning that the odds of a case being exposed to dental radiographs were 1.17 times the odds of a control being exposed to dental radiographs.

Strengths and limitations

Case-control studies have several strengths. The efficiency of the retrospective design and the ability to examine the association of multiple exposures and an outcome of interest, even if the outcome is rare, make them suitable as hypothesis-generating studies. In addition, there are some circumstances where a direct prospective observation from exposure to outcome would take several decades (e.g., alcohol consumption and cancer). Case-control studies can also provide evidence to support a potential exposure-outcome association using relatively few subjects compared to other prospective designs. While in general cohort studies would require sample sizes of thousands of subjects, case-control studies can be well conducted with only hundreds of participants, which makes them efficient in studying associations between exposures and infrequent outcomes (e.g., bacillary epithelium angiomatosis). Case-control studies also have major limitations. Investigators must exert tremendous effort to identify cases (participants with the outcome of interest). Although participants can provide information on multiple exposures that occurred in the past simultaneously, by design, only one outcome can be studied at a time. This is a key weakness compared to other analytical observational study designs or randomized controlled trials, which allow for the exploration of the effect of an exposure on multiple outcomes simultaneously. Another major limitation of case-control studies is that they are highly susceptible to many sources of bias. The distinctive selection of cases and controls and the retrospective nature of the determination of the exposure are among the most serious issues threatening the validity of case-control studies. Case-control studies play an important role in epidemiology, but their conclusions should be interpreted cautiously and mostly used as hypothesis-generating findings.

The price of two cars and the case-control study design

To know the price of an SUV, a car buyer has visited two dealerships in the neighborhood. At the first dealership, the cost of last year's SUV, including all add-on features, was $37,000 (car 1 = control). At the second dealership, however, the price of the same vehicle with the same add-on features and mileage was only $25,000 (car 2= case). How is it possible that two SUV models so similar have very different prices? Before making a final offer, the car buyer, skeptical of the price at the second dealership, brought along a friend who knows everything about cars. The friend asked several questions to the seller, who provided all the information about the car without indicating the reason for the large price discrepancy. Then, the friend examined the car and noticed several unequivocal signs that the SUV from the second dealership had been involved in a collision (exposed), while the SUV from the first dealership had not been involved in a collision (unexposed). They concluded that the collision was likely the reason for the price difference.

Selected readings

Brignardello-Petersen R, Carrasco-Labra A, Glick M, Guyatt GH, Azarpazhooh A. A practical approach to evidence-based dentistry: IV: how to use an article about harm. *J Am Dent Assoc.* 2015 Feb;146(2):94–101.e1.

Schulz KF, Grimes DA. Case-control studies: research in reverse. *Lancet.* 2002 Feb 2;359(9304):431–434.

Sedgwick P. Bias in observational study designs: case-control studies. *BMJ.* 2015 Jan 30;350:h560.

Sedgwick P. Case-control studies: advantages and disadvantages. *BMJ.* 2014 Jan 3;348:f7707.

17

Understanding and interpreting a cohort study

Cohort studies are classic types of epidemiological designs. The most important feature distinguishing a cohort study from other *observational studies* is temporality. In a cohort study design, it is possible to determine that an exposure has occurred prior to an *outcome*. A cohort is a group of individuals who share specific characteristics (e.g., live in the same geographic area, are a similar age, work in the same office building) and are followed to determine if a specific outcome (e.g., a disease) can be predicted based on the existence a particular exposure (e.g., potential *risk factor*). The ability to predict the effect of these exposures on the onset of disease provides the basis for prevention at both individual and *population* levels.

Both cohort study designs and *randomized controlled trials* (RCT) are prospective in nature and provide evidence about the temporal association between an exposure and an outcome of interest. The key distinction between cohort studies and RCT designs is that an RCT is an *experimental study* where investigators deliberately and randomly allocate the exposure to one or more experimental interventions (Chapter 18). In contrast, a cohort study is an observational study where researchers do not choose which participants experience an exposure. Since participants are deliberately and randomly allocated to the experimental and control arms in an RCT, the influence of *confounding* is minimized and researchers can make stronger arguments for causal inferences than can be made with cohort studies (Chapter 12). The ability to make causal inferences in an RCT is a benefit of this study design. However, RCTs are not helpful when studying the effects of potentially harmful exposures or interventions. Even if a research question about harm has a sound rationale and represents a knowledge gap, it would be unethical to randomly assign participants to be exposed to such harm. A second limitation is that RCTs often include a narrow and high-risk population to ensure that if no effect is apparent in this population, others would be unlikely to benefit from the new treatment. The problem with this approach is that trials conducted under such a premise may not be generalizable or applicable to a larger group of individuals or populations. Cohort studies offer several aspects that overcome these issues. They can be conducted on a large population and allow for examining the effect of an exposure on an outcome without intentionally assigning participants to exposures of interest.

Types of cohort study designs

Prospective and retrospective or historical cohort studies are frequently reported in the research literature. In prospective cohort studies, investigators define a priori how the exposure of interest, risk factors, and outcomes will be measured, plan calibration training for those in charge of

Statistics for Dental Clinicians, First Edition. Michael Glick, Alonso Carrasco-Labra, and Olivia Urquhart.
© 2024 John Wiley & Sons, Inc. Published 2024 by John Wiley & Sons, Inc.

measuring variables and consult the literature to obtain the best available evidence regarding potential *confounders* to measure and adjust for in designing the study and the analysis. Since investigators collect data as the study is conducted, this design can also be called a *concurrent cohort study*. The possibility to plan and implement rigorous data quality assurance, the ability to plan, measure, and adjust for confounding variables, and the possibility to accurately estimate the magnitude and length of exposure that resulted in the outcomes of interest are some of the main advantages of concurrent cohort studies.

The second type of study design is based on *retrospective or historical cohorts*. In this design, investigators take advantage of data already available and collected in the past. In most situations, these data were collected for purposes other than the study at hand; these data precede or are nonconcurrent with the conduct of the study. This is the reason retrospective cohort studies are also called *nonconcurrent cohort studies*. This design has several advantages. The time between the exposure(s) and the outcome occurred in the past, which provides efficiency (the researcher does not need to wait for an outcome to occur and observe study participants for long periods) and makes the study less resource-intensive (the data have already been collected) than a prospective design. For example, using a carefully curated national registry with preexisting data to construct a retrospective cohort allows investigators to work with low rates of missing participant data. The major downside of a retrospective cohort design is that the data were seldom collected for the purposes of the study at hand; also, the methods and consistency for measuring exposures and outcomes cannot always be ensured and may not be optimal for the particular study. Data entry for large population-level databases is often performed by numerous institutions and centers and collected by individuals with different levels of training and expertise, leading to inconsistencies in the application of diagnostic criteria, risk factor assessment, and outcome measures. In addition, some potential confounding variables that need to be controlled for in the analysis may not have been measured, reducing the credibility of any identified association.

Using the prospective and retrospective terminology to refer to cohort studies often creates confusion with other designs, such as case-control studies, which are retrospective in nature (Chapter 16). Whether investigators collected exposures and outcomes prospectively (i.e., concurrently) or took advantage of large preexisting patient databases to assemble a cohort (i.e., nonconcurrently), both designs allow for determining that exposures occurred or risk factors were present before the outcome of interest. This allows for establishing the temporal sequence from exposure to outcome. A third subtype of cohort study combines elements of both prospective and retrospective cohorts, for example, by using a retrospective (nonconcurrent) or historical unexposed group and a prospective (concurrent) exposed group (Figure 17.1).

Selection of the study population

An essential feature of a cohort study is the presence of exposed and unexposed groups of participants to measure the *incidence* of the outcome of interest. One way to create these groups is, by design, to enroll people based on whether they have or have not experienced the exposure. In other words, exposure status is an eligibility criterion to enter the study. Another option is to identify a group of people for the study before any of them have had the opportunity of being exposed to the risk factor of interest but who share a common characteristic; maybe they all live in the same zip code or reside in a specific setting, such as a nursing home. Clinical examinations and other measures required to distinguish the exposed from the unexposed are implemented while the

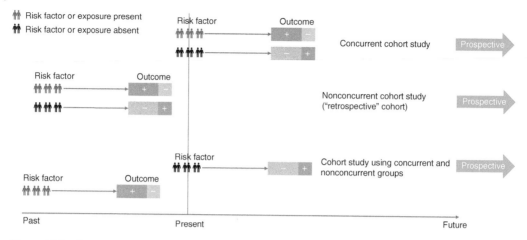

Figure 17.1   Three types of cohort study designs and temporality. Blue horizontal arrows represent a timeline from past to future. The vertical blue line represents the present time. Red figures depict individuals exposed to a risk factor of interest while black figures depict individuals unexposed to a risk factor of interest. A green box with a + sign reflects the presence of an outcome of interest while a yellow box with a - sign reflects the absence of an outcome of interest. Risk factors and outcomes are measured simultaneously in this type of design. The blue arrows pointing to the future (to the right) illustrate the prospective aspect of the study design, i.e., the assessment of the association of interest starts from exposed and unexposed individuals and follow up prospectively to determine the presence or absence of an outcome.

participants are already enrolled in the study. Regardless of the recruitment strategy, the result is the same—for analysis, recruited individuals are split into exposed and unexposed groups.

Measuring exposures

When using the word *exposure*, investigators refer to several factors that correspond to any characteristic or attribute of a participant or any external agent that can determine a person's health or the presence or absence of disease. For example, age, sex, race/ethnicity, genetics, and metabolism are intrinsic factors. External or environmental factors can include coming in contact with a microorganism, exposure to pollution and contaminating agents, smoking, and dietary habits. Measuring exposure is not always straightforward. For some exposures, it is relatively easy to identify their timing and intensity. For example, it would be easy to quantify the amount of radiation exposure for individuals in proximity to a nuclear power plant accident on a specific calendar day and time using a reliable instrument. Other exposures or risk factors, for example, socioeconomic status, contain several layers of complexity, including multiple environmental and behavioral factors, that are difficult to separate and study individually. Exposures can also be fixed over time or vary as time passes. People tend to modify their dietary habits over their lifetime, may migrate to another country or continent, or may intermittently quit and resume smoking. These are called individual time-dependent exposures as they vary over time. Other exposures, for example, regular weather fluctuations throughout a year, the amount of pollutants in the air in a particular geographic area, and the inclusion of new therapeutic interventions at a health system level, represent external time-dependent exposures. These factors fluctuate over time and affect entire populations.

Exposures can be defined as *quantitative* (e.g., *continuous*) or *qualitative* (e.g., *categorical*) variables. Measuring exposures that are quantitative in nature requires calibrated equipment or instruments, such as a sphygmomanometer or a glucose monitor, to determine physiological factors or the use of reliable and valid questionnaires for patient-reported outcome measures (Chapter 14). Qualitative exposures also require the use of standardized questionnaires and clinical examinations with clear operational definitions (e.g., current smoker, never a smoker, ex-smoker). All these measures require the use of calibrated equipment or research personnel previously trained to achieve high levels of *intra- and inter-rater reliability* (Chapter 14).

Measuring outcome frequency

Unlike *cross-sectional studies* (Chapter 15), which primarily report prevalence estimates, in cohort studies, when the outcome of interest is dichotomous, two common measures for the frequency can be calculated: the *cumulative incidence* and the *incidence rate*. These measures are quotients and include in the numerator the number of individuals in the study who developed the outcome of interest. The data in the numerator reflect the prospective nature of cohort studies, as the outcomes are counted and accumulated as the study progresses. Not everyone in the study would experience the outcome, yet the entire study population should be "at risk," which is reflected in the denominator of the estimates. When the number in the denominator is the population without the disease at baseline (population at risk), the resulting measure of disease frequency is called cumulative incidence or *incidence proportion*. Investigators can also account for unforeseeable events that prevent them from observing the outcome of an individual in the study as time passes, for example, a participant moving to another city who is lost to follow-up or death for reasons unrelated to the study purpose. Using a measure called *person-time* at risk allows accounting for the disease-free time that a participant contributed to the study from baseline to (1) the timepoint when the outcome of interest occurred, (2) the timepoint when the study ends and the outcome did not yet occur (i.e., *censoring*) (Chapter 8), or (3) the timepoint when a person is considered lost to follow-up. The person-time at risk is a rate and includes in the denominator a combination of at-risk time periods, often using year as a unit, for every participant in the study. For example, an individual in a 10-year cohort study who completes the follow-up without experiencing the outcome will contribute with 10 person-years.

An application of the concepts of cumulative incidence and incidence rate is presented in the following study. A hypothetical cohort study including 100 individuals followed up for two years showed an incidence of five new cases per year. The cumulative incidence was 10 out of 100, or 10%, after two years of follow-up (Appendix 1, Equation 17.1). The incidence rate takes into account that the participants who had the outcome of interest during year 1 (5 participants in this example) do not have the chance of experiencing the outcome during year 2 and hence are excluded from the denominator for the calculation of person-year at risk for year 2. Therefore, the incidence rate is 0.052 or 5.2 per 100 person-years (Appendix 1, Equation 17.2).

Measures of association

Besides the measures of disease frequency presented above (cumulative incidence and incidence rate), measures of association can help to compare two groups in a cohort study using one of two mathematical operators: subtraction (absolute measures) or division (relative measures). The *risk difference*, *risk ratio* or *relative risk*, the *odds ratio* (Chapter 2), and the *hazard ratio* (Chapter 8) are examples of these types of measures. Another example of these measures is the *rate ratio* (*incidence density ratio*), which is a measure of association that represents the ratio of the incidence rate in an exposed group and the incidence rate in the unexposed group.

Bias in cohort studies

Bias or systematic error refers to anomalies in the identification and recruitment of participants, inaccuracies in the measurement of exposures or risk factors and outcomes, or misguided presentations of study findings that produce a deviation from the truth (Chapter 13). Observational studies, including cohort studies, are prone to three main types of biases: *selection bias*, *information bias*, and confounding.

Selection bias

This is a broad group of biases that result in a cohort study sample that differs from the population from which it was initially drawn. Selection bias can be minimized by implementing an appropriate sampling framework, including in the study participants who resemble the general population, and minimizing loss to follow-up.

Nonparticipation and nonresponse

Investigators taking a sample from the population of interest will inevitably confront some eligible people who decline the invitation to participate (nonparticipation). Researchers may also encounter potentially eligible people who ignore the invitation (nonresponse). This phenomenon would not necessarily be a source of bias unless those refusing participation or ignoring the invitation are more likely to be exposed or have the risk factor and the subsequent outcome compared to those who accepted the invitation or responded to the participation request. If this is the case, the cohort study results would be prone to underestimate an association between exposure and outcome compared to the general population. It is difficult to determine the extension of this type of bias given that information regarding those refusing participation or not responding is inaccessible to the investigators.

Loss to follow-up or attrition bias

The risk of losing participants to follow-up is high in long-term, large-cohort studies, and researchers dedicate extensive effort to minimize this issue. *Attrition bias* is of concern when the reason for loss to follow-up is related to the exposure or the outcome of interest. For example, if people who experience or have a high risk of experiencing the outcome are more prone to leave the study, and those who leave the study are systematically different from those remaining in the study, the estimate of the association between exposure/nonexposure and the outcome will be distorted.

Information bias: Dissimilar information between exposed and unexposed participants

This type of bias can happen when the exposure or outcome is incorrectly identified or measured by investigators, intentionally or unintentionally, dedicating differential efforts to collecting data among exposed versus unexposed participants. If these issues have the same chance of happening, regardless of whether individuals are exposed or unexposed and regardless of whether they experience the outcome or not, it is known as *nondifferential misclassification bias*. For example, if mortality records containing billing codes are used to ascertain an outcome, they may contain mistakes, and the frequency of these mistakes will not depend on whether or not someone was exposed or unexposed. Alternatively, if this misclassification of the exposure or outcome depends on the outcome and exposure status, respectively, *differential misclassification bias* will occur. Sometimes the study design, for example, a nonconcurrent cohort study (a retrospective cohort), may determine better data availability and quality among the exposed compared to unexposed individuals. Both types of misclassification can distort research findings of an association between exposure and outcome. An example of this type of bias occurs when the investigators measuring the outcome of interest are aware of the exposure status of the participants. Some outcomes like death, a cardiovascular event, tooth loss, surgical site infection, or detachment of a crown are straightforward to observe and measure, with little to no space for subjective interpretation. Other outcomes, like facial swelling measured with a qualitative scale, caries progression, or the healing status of an oral lesion, are more subjective and prone to be affected by the researcher's awareness of the exposure status of the participant. Investigators knowing the hypothesis being tested can protect themselves from this bias by including in the study design a masking strategy. Masking, also known as *blinding*, can minimize the effect of this bias not only for the investigators ascertaining the outcome of interest but also for other study personnel, including clinicians and biostatisticians.

Confounding

Confounding is one of the most important issues affecting the validity of *cohort* studies, as the inability to control or adjust for *confounding variables* results in a distortion of the potential association under investigation. *Specification* (sometimes also called restriction), *stratification*, *propensity score*, and *multivariable regression* analysis are some strategies used by investigators to minimize the impact of confounding variables (Chapter 11).

Strengths and limitations

The most significant strength of a cohort study is that it allows for the estimation of incidence, the frequency or rate of new cases of a disease, or the presence of an outcome of interest over time. The prospective nature of a cohort study, with the ascertainment of the outcome always occurring after the ascertainment of the exposure, makes the time sequence informative for making causal inferences. A third important strength is that cohort studies are efficient in studying the effect of multiple exposures or risk factors on an outcome while at the same time allowing for the assessment of the association between a single exposure or risk factor on multiple outcomes. Cohort studies also have important limitations, many common to other observational study designs. Although investigators can implement methodological and statistical strategies to minimize the effect of confounding, there is still a possibility of residual confounding. In addition, cohort studies are expensive to conduct and inefficient when the outcome of interest is infrequent. They are better suited for continuous outcomes or for easy-to-measure dichotomous outcomes with a relatively short timeframe between exposure and outcome.

A house on the beach, Jeep corrosion, and a rusty undercarriage

A long time ago, my brother and I each wanted to buy a Jeep. After looking at our options, we chose the same brand and Jeep model and we got two identical vehicles. Aware of my brother's home location on a coastline in Florida, we thought about whether the salt from seawater (exposure to seawater) would result in corrosion and a rusty undercarriage for his Jeep (outcome). He drove from where I live, Atlanta (nonexposure to seawater), to his place in Florida.

Ten years passed (follow-up) before I drove from Atlanta to Florida to visit my brother. I decided to compare side by side how much corrosion and rust his Jeep had compared to mine. As expected, his Jeep had clear signs of damage easily associated with the effect of seawater on the chassis. My Jeep had never been exposed to seawater and did not present the same signs of corrosion. After ten years of follow-up, I concluded that seawater is a risk factor for a rusty Jeep's undercarriage.

Suggested readings

Grimes DA, Schultz KF. Cohort studies: marching towards outcomes. *Lancet.* 2002;359:341–345.

McNamee R. Confounding and confounders. *Occup Environ Med.* 2003 Mar;60(3):227–234; quiz 164, 234.

Sedgwick P. Bias in observational study designs: prospective cohort studies. *BMJ.* 2014 Dec 19;349:g7731.

Sedgwick P. Estimating the population at risk. *BMJ.* 2012;345:e6859.

Wang X, Kattan MW. Cohort studies: design, analysis, and reporting. *Chest.* 2020 Jul;158(1S):S72–S78.

18

Understanding and interpreting a randomized controlled trial

Understanding aspects of how to plan and conduct a study, including a *randomized controlled trial* (RCT), will help to inform clinical practice. A *clinical trial* is a prospective *experimental study* involving human subjects that compares the *effect* of one or more *interventions* with that in a *control group* where all *variables* that may affect or influence the *outcomes* other than the intervention are controlled or held constant. Although all participants may not enter the trial at the same time, they are all followed for a similar timeframe, between time zero (i.e., baseline) and follow-up completion (i.e., end of the study). Study designs that are retrospective in nature, such as *case-control studies*, are not classified as clinical trials (Chapter 16). Neither are *cohort study* designs, which may use existing clinical records that contain information collected in the past linking an intervention to an *outcome* (Chapter 17). These designs do not meet the criteria to be called clinical trials, as the investigators do not directly observe the effect of the intervention on the participants prospectively from baseline to follow-up. Additionally, investigators cannot control or influence the actions of the participants in these studies. Controlling variables (e.g., pharmacological interventions or behaviors that may affect the study results) is an important element of a clinical trial in order to attribute observed effects solely to the intervention of interest to the researcher.

An RCT is a type of clinical trial in which investigators are interested in the effect of an *exposure* (an intervention) on outcomes. What sets RCTs apart from *observational studies* is the act of deliberately randomizing the allocation of the intervention to participants in the study. The main advantage of well-conducted RCTs over observational studies (*cross-sectional*, case-control, and cohort studies) (Chapter 15, 16, and 17) is their ability to provide evidence of causality. This advantage resides in the temporal sequence of administering an intervention before observing its effect (Figure 18.1). The benefit of the manner in which participants are allocated into groups (e.g., intervention and control groups) is that the influence of *confounding* is minimized (Chapter 12). Confounding is a phenomenon often encountered when conducting observational studies that distorts the association being studied. The purpose of randomly allocating participants to *study arms* (receiving or not receiving the intervention) is for the groups to be comparable in their distribution of *prognostic factors*—any factor except the intervention that may influence the outcome—and known and unknown *confounders* (Figure 18.2). Achieving and maintaining the balance of prognostic factors between study arms throughout the study provides confidence that the appropriate methodological norms were followed and that any observed *treatment effect* can be attributed to the intervention and not to *bias* or confounding (Chapters 12 and 13).

Statistics for Dental Clinicians, First Edition. Michael Glick, Alonso Carrasco-Labra, and Olivia Urquhart.
© 2024 John Wiley & Sons, Inc. Published 2024 by John Wiley & Sons, Inc.

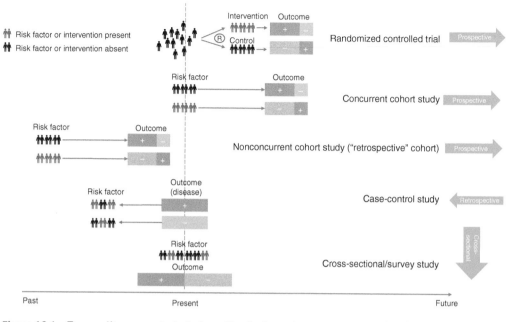

Figure 18.1 Temporality across study designs. Blue horizontal arrows represent timelines. The vertical dashed blue line represents the present time. Red figures depict individuals exposed to an intervention or risk factor of interest, while black figures depict individuals unexposed to an intervention or risk factor of interest. A green box with a + sign reflects the presence of an outcome of interest, while a yellow box with a - sign reflects the absence of an outcome of interest. The blue arrows pointing to the future (to the right) illustrate the prospective aspect of the study design, i.e., the assessment of the association of interest starts from exposed and unexposed individuals and follow up prospectively to determine the presence or absence of an outcome or disease of interest. The blue arrows pointing to the past (to the left) illustrate the retrospective aspect of the study design, i.e., the assessment of the association of interest starts from people with and without the outcome or disease of interest and retrospectively examines whether they were exposed or unexposed to a risk factor. The absence of blue arrows (cross-sectional/survey study) represents the measurement of risk factors and outcome or disease of interest simultaneously.

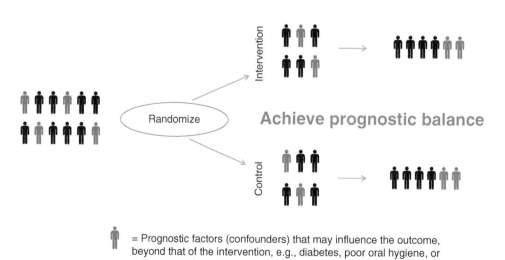

Figure 18.2 The purpose of randomization in a randomized controlled trial.

Study arms

Both observational (e.g., case-control studies, cohort studies) and experimental studies, such as RCTs, aim to quantify associations between exposures or interventions and outcomes. In RCTs, study participants are randomly divided into two or more groups—the intervention group(s) and the control group. These groups are commonly referred to as study arms. The intervention group, or intervention arm, usually receives or is subjected to an active intervention(s) (e.g., an antibiotic, surgery, fluoride rinse), while the control group can consist of a placebo, where the formulation, look, feel, smell, and taste are similar to the intervention but does not contain the active ingredient, another type of intervention for an active comparison, or no intervention at all. An active comparison could be a different formulation of a tooth whitener. In surgical RCTs, a placebo group can consist of participants who underwent a sham surgery (a surgical procedure up to the point of incision) to mimic active surgery.

Type of outcomes

Outcomes are constructs or variables of interest in a research study that are speculated to be affected by another variable, such as a clinical intervention or an exposure. *Measures of association* quantify the magnitude of an association or a treatment effect between study groups (Chapter 2). These measures inform which interventions may be the most effective in a clinical setting and serve as the basis for clinical decision making.

Before the initiation of an RCT, a set of outcomes to be recorded for each participant at specified time points during the study is specified. However, not all outcomes are created equal. Outcomes most useful for clinical decision making are those where a patient's values, what the patient cares about, are addressed. Such outcomes are referred to as *patient-important outcomes*. For example, in a study comparing root canal therapy to extractions and subsequent placement of an implant, patients may care most about outcomes such as number of procedures, aesthetics, time, or cost. A similar concept is a *patient-reported outcome measures*, which captures the patient's subjective reported health status and wellbeing through their experiences (Chapter 14).

When researchers set out to produce evidence of preliminary *efficacy* of an intervention they sometimes select *surrogate outcomes* for their study, or outcomes that are precursors, predictors, or proxies of clinician- or patient-important outcomes. These outcomes typically take less time to observe than patient-important outcomes so researchers may extrapolate them to the patient-important outcomes that typically require more time to observe. Importantly, surrogate markers may not correctly reflect a clinical outcome. The statistical methods available to extrapolate surrogate outcomes to patient-important outcomes are of questionable utility. Consider a hypothetical study comparing the effectiveness of two sealant types. The researcher measures the difference in the *Streptococcus mutans* bacteria level between caries-free participants who received sealant A and those who received sealant B. The patient-important outcome is advanced carious lesions, but the researchers chose to instead measure *Streptococcus mutans* bacteria, a surrogate outcome, because they need to finish their study in six months and advanced carious lesions take much longer to develop. The chosen surrogate markers may not reflect a clinical outcome. For example, how well an elevated *Streptococcus mutans* level can predict the development of advanced carious lesions may be unknown. Not everyone with elevated levels of bacteria will develop advanced caries, and conversely individuals with low bacteria levels may still develop them.

Investigators may identify more than one critical or primary outcome to collect in their study and can combine two or more outcomes into a single outcome—a *composite outcome*. Composite outcomes can be advantageous because they offer a greater chance of observing *events* when they are combined than if assessed separately. This is advantageous from a resource perspective as the investigator can use a smaller sample size when they combine outcomes—rather than measuring each outcome separately—without sacrificing statistical power (Chapter 7). One of the major drawbacks of using composite outcome measures is the possibility of observing an effect in the composite outcome that contradicts the observed effect in individual outcomes. In a hypothetical study, 200 people are randomized equally into a group that will take low-dose aspirin daily and a group that will not. After five years, a composite outcome of experiencing either stroke or death was measured for each study participant. The relative risk (RR) of experiencing a stroke or death in the aspirin group (16 events of stroke or death) compared to the no aspirin group (26 events of stroke or death) was 0.62 (Chapter 2), so the researcher can conclude that aspirin reduces the risk of stroke and death by 38% (Appendix 1, Equation 18.1a; Table 18.1a). If the investigator were to have looked at stroke and death separately (Tables 18.1b, 18.1c), the conclusions would have been different. Most of the 16 and 26 events tabulated in the composite outcome could be attributed to people who had strokes. Only one person in each group passed away. The RR for the outcome death was 1.00 (Appendix 1, Equation 18.1b), meaning that the risk of death was the same between the two groups. The RR for the outcome stroke was 0.60 (Appendix 1, Equation 18.1c), very similar to that for the composite outcome. Concluding that aspirin reduces the risk of experiencing stroke or dying by 38% would be a misleading or incomplete picture of the underlying truth because the risk of death was the same between the two groups. This is an extreme example of how a composite outcome can produce misleading conclusions.

Table 18.1a   Relative risk for the composite outcome stroke or death.

		Outcome		
		Stroke or death	**No stroke or death**	**Absolute risk**
Intervention	Aspirin (100)	15 strokes + 1 death = 16	84	16/100 = 0.16
	No aspirin (100)	25 strokes + 1 death = 26	74	26/100 = 0.26

Relative risk	0.16/0.26 = 0.62

Table 18.1b   Relative risk for the outcome stroke.

		Outcome		
		Stroke	**No stroke**	**Absolute risk**
Intervention	Aspirin (100)	15	85	15/100 = 0.15
	No aspirin (100)	25	75	25/100 = 0.25

Relative risk	0.15/0.25 = 0.60

Table 18.1c Relative risk for the outcome death.

		Outcome		
		Death	No death	Absolute risk
Intervention	Aspirin (100)	1	99	$1/100 = 0.01$
	No aspirin (100)	1	99	$1/100 = 0.01$
		Relative risk		$0.01/0.01 = 1.00$

Methodological strategies in randomized controlled trials

In the context of an RCT, a *random sequence* is a list of randomly generated numbers that indicates which study arm study participants will be allocated to. Once a random sequence is generated, different methods are used to guard or conceal the randomization sequence from the study personnel responsible for enrolling patients. Such an approach is known as *allocation concealment* and is employed to eliminate the possibility that those enrolling patients can manipulate and unduly influence the randomization process (selection bias). Tampering with the randomization sequence can threaten its integrity and hence the balance of prognostic factors between groups. Including treatment assignments in consecutively-opened sealed opaque envelopes and labeling pill bottles with anonymized codes are two ways to conceal the treatment allocation. Central randomization is another method whereby the investigator contacts a third-party call center. The call center is the keeper of the randomization sequence and will notify the investigator which study arm the next study participant enrolled in trial should be allocated to.

Once the study participant is assigned to a treatment arm, it is important that those involved in the study conduct are blinded about which treatment arm the participants were allocated to. People who should be blinded include health care providers, study participants, outcome assessors, data analysts, and personnel interpreting the results. Blinding ensures that study participants and personnel don't change their behavior in a way that could affect the study results. For instance, if a participant knows they were allocated to a placebo, they may take other remedies or treatments to help improve their condition with the knowledge that they currently aren't using any active medication. Further, if study personnel or patients self-report a subjective outcome (e.g., trismus, pain on a visual analog scale, oral-health-related quality of life) know the treatment received, their assessments of the outcome may be subconsciously influenced by this knowledge.

Nonadherence to study protocol

Measures of association like RRs, odds ratios, and mean differences quantify the effect of an intervention compared to a control group in an RCT (Chapter 2). During the conduct of an RCT, some study participants will not adhere to their randomly allocated protocol. In some cases, they won't take their allocated intervention or may take the intervention intended for participants in another study arm. A way to handle this when calculating measures of association is to conduct an *intention-to-treat analysis*, where those who didn't adhere to the intervention are nevertheless analyzed in the group they were randomized to. In other words, the fact that they switched groups or didn't take the intervention they were allocated to is ignored (Figure 18.3). This approach is advantageous because it maintains the

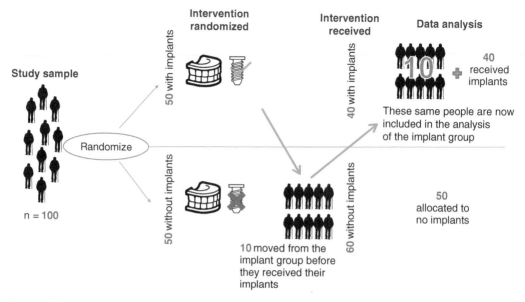

Figure 18.3 Intention-to-treat analysis.

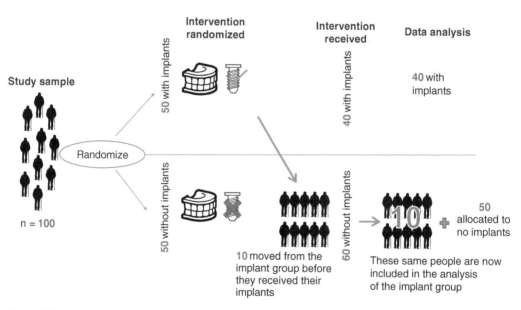

Figure 18.4 As treated analysis.

randomized allocation of the study participants and in turn the *prognostic balance* between study arms. Another way to manage this issue is to conduct an *as-treated analysis*, where study participants are analyzed in the group according to the intervention they actually received or took (Figure 18.4). A third option to address the issue is to conduct a *naïve per-protocol analysis* and include in the analysis participants who adhered to the study arm they were allocated to (Figure 18.5). All three options are accompanied by drawbacks. One issue with intention-to-treat analysis is that harmful outcomes will appear to be less harmful than they actually are. Additionally, both the second and third options are problematic because they break the original randomization sequence, which may result in an imbalance in prognostic factors between groups.

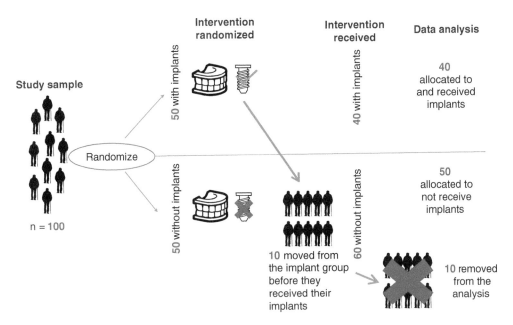

Figure 18.5 Naïve per-protocol analysis.

Missing data

Another threat to the *validity* of an RCT is having participants dropping out or missing their follow-up visit. One approach to assess the impact of missing data on the study results is to pretend that everyone who was lost in the intervention arm experienced the event of interest for the outcome and everyone who was lost in the control arm did not—*worst-case scenario analysis*. In hypothetical study A, out of 100 study participants in the intervention group, 20 experienced a harmful outcome and 2 were lost to follow-up, while out of the 100 study participants in the control group, 40 experienced the harmful outcome and 2 were lost to follow-up. If the 4 people lost to follow-up were ignored in the analysis, the RR would be 0.50 (Appendix 1, Equation 18.2a, Table 18.2). If the investigators were to pretend that the 2 people in the intervention group who were lost experienced the negative outcome and the 2 people lost in the control group did not, the RR would be 0.55 (Appendix 1, Equation 18.2a, Table 18.2). This worst-case scenario estimate, 0.55, is more

Table 18.2 Impact of missing participant data in treatment effect estimates.

	Study A		Study B	
	Intervention	Control	Intervention	Control
No. of participants included in the study	100	100	100	100
No. of participants lost to follow-up (%)	2 (2)	2 (2)	2 (2)	2 (2)
No. of events: alveolar osteitis (%)	20 (20)	40 (40)	2 (2)	4 (4)
Effect ignoring lost to follow-up	RR: 0.20/0.40 = 0.50		RR: 0.02/0.04 = 0.50	
Effect worst-case scenario	RR: 0.22/0.40 = 0.55		RR: 0.04/0.04 = 1.0	

RR: relative risk.

conservative, albeit just by 5%, than the estimate ignoring those lost (0.50) as it underestimates the treatment effect—brings it closer to 1 (no difference)—in the risk between the groups. In study A, the observed events were common, occurring in 20% and 40% of the participants in each study arm respectively. Now, consider study B, where the observed events were rare, occurring in only 2% and 4% of study participants in the intervention and control arms, respectively. Like study A, in study B 2 study participants were lost in each group. When lost to follow-up is ignored, the RR in this case is still 0.50 (Appendix 1, Equation 18.2b, Table 18.2), but when the worst-case scenario assumes that the 2 people lost in the intervention group experienced the harmful outcome, the RR is 1.0 (Appendix 1, Equation 18.2b; Table 18.2). Issues of missing data can distort the study results, which is of particular concern when the events of an outcome are rare.

Subgroup analysis or effect modification

Clinicians aim to personalize treatment options for their patients. This can be accomplished by distinguishing patients who would benefit the most from an intervention (a treatment option) from those who would benefit the least. In the planning phases of an RCT, investigators can hypothesize that a treatment may be more effective in some study participants compared to others. These differences in effect could be derived from the participant demographics, the clinical presentation of disease, or the severity or type of disease. *Subgroup analysis* can test these hypotheses (Chapter 5). Consider a hypothetical study where a new oncology treatment is compared to an existing one. The investigators hypothesize that a new treatment will be more effective in reducing the chance of recurrence of a cancerous lesion compared to an existing treatment and calculated an RR of 0.25 (95% CI: 0.19 to 0.33) (Appendix 1, Equation 18.3a and 18.3b), meaning that the new treatment reduced the chance of the cancerous lesion reoccurring by 75% (Table 18.3a) (ranging from an 81% to 67% reduction).

Additionally, considering the biological process of the cancerous lesion, the investigators also hypothesized that the new treatment would be more effective in reducing the risk of reoccurrence of cancerous lesions with mutation A compared to mutation B. The investigators separated all of the study participants into two groups, subgroup A, comprising all participants with mutation A, and subgroup B, comprising all participants with mutation B, and calculated an RR and 95% confidence interval (CI) for each group. The RRs were 0.10 (95% CI: 0.04 to 0.24) (Table 18.3b; Appendix 1,

Table 18.3a Relative risk for the primary analysis (n = 500).

		Outcomes		
		Cancerous lesion reoccurrence	No cancerous lesion reoccurrence	Absolute risk
Intervention	New oncology treatment (500)	50	450	50/500 = 0.10
	Existing oncology treatment (500)	200	300	200/500 = 0.40

Relative risk	0.25 (95% CI: 0.19 to 0.33)

Table 18.3b   Relative risk for the subgroup, all study participants with mutation A (n=250).

		Outcomes		
		Cancerous lesion reoccurrence	**No cancerous lesion reoccurrence**	**Absolute risk**
Intervention	New oncology treatment (125)	5	120	5/125 = 0.04
	Existing oncology treatment (125)	50	75	50/125 = 0.40

Relative risk	0.10 (95% CI: 0.04 to 0.24)

Table 18.3c   Relative risk for the subgroup, all study participants with mutation B (n=250).

		Outcomes		
		Cancerous lesion reoccurrence	**No cancerous lesion reoccurrence**	**Absolute risk**
Intervention	New oncology treatment (125)	20	105	20/125 = 0.16
	Existing oncology treatment (125)	50	75	50/125 = 0.40

Relative risk	0.40 (95% CI: 0.25 to 0.63)

Equation 18.3c and 18.3d) in group A and 0.40 (95% CI: 0.25 to 0.63) (Table 18.3c; Appendix 1, Equation 18.3e and 18.3f) in group B. The CIs between the two subgroups do not overlap (Chapter 6) and the p-value for the subgroup analysis is 0.01, meaning that there is a statistically significant difference in the treatment effect between study participants with mutation A compared to mutation B (Chapter 5).

How trustworthy a subgroup analysis is depends on the investigators defining the variables and hypothesizing the direction and magnitude of the subgroup effect a priori (during the study planning phase). If these analyses are not preplanned, the investigators, especially in the face of negative results (statistically nonsignificant findings) in their main analysis, may look for subgroup effects after they've analyzed the data. Second, subgroup analyses should be interpreted with caution, as dividing the study sample into subgroups dilutes the sample size, which impacts the study power (1 − type II error) (Chapter 7). This reduction in power means that differences in subgroups may exist, but the statistical test for subgroup effects may not be able to detect such a difference. Last, subgroup analyses should be few in number, as the more subgroup analyses the investigator performs, the more likely they will find a statistically significant difference in a given subgroup just by chance (type I error) (Chapter 7).

A few additional notes

- *Comparative effectiveness* research is focused on the generation of data (e.g., using RCTs) and synthesis (Chapter 19) of evidence to inform the benefits and harms of alternatives to manage and prevent clinical conditions.
- There are other types of clinical trials where study participants are not randomized. They are known as nonrandomized or quasi-randomized clinical trials. In these studies, the research participants are allocated to groups, but the allocation is nonrandom. For example, patients entering a clinic in the evening are allocated to study arm 1, those in the morning and afternoon to study arm 2. This is not truly a random method of allocating study participants because evening patients may be different from morning and afternoon patients. Other pseudo-methods include allocating patients by their area code or their patient ID number.
- Special types of randomized controlled trial designs: When individual people are randomized to study arms, this is referred to as a *parallel RCT*. However, there are many variations to parallel RCTs. One common example is a *cluster RCT*, where instead of individual people being randomized to groups, clusters or groups are randomized to the study arms. In other words, the unit of randomization is not an individual person but rather a group like a classroom, hospital, or family. Since the individuals within each group may be similar, when analyzing the data from these RCTs, these similarities or nonindependence must be accounted for. Another common subtype of RCT encountered in the oral health literature is called a *split-body RCT* (or split-mouth RCT). Instead of randomizing individual humans to study arms, their individual body parts are randomized. For example, teeth in different quadrants of the mouth in the same individual can be randomized to a given study arm. Such studies are advantageous because each person acts as their own control group with the sole difference between the study arms being the selected body part, in our example, quadrant of the mouth. However, the same data analysis considerations apply as in cluster RCTs. Other RCTs encountered in the literature include adaptive, stepped wedge, wait list, factorial, and n-of-1.
- Randomization of study participants into groups in RCTs to achieve prognostic balance is conceptually similar to matching in observational studies. Randomization in an RCT accounts for known and unknown confounders, whereas matching only accounts for known confounders (Chapter 12 and 13).
- *Simple randomization* is the most straightforward method for randomizing study participants and involves the creation of just one random sequence of numbers. This can be achieved by tossing a fair coin, where heads means the person is allocated to the treatment group, tails the control group. More sophisticated ways include referencing a random number table or generating a random number sequence from a computer program. These methods work fairly well when the sample size is large, but when the sample size is small, by chance the random sequence may allocate many more people to one study arm compared to another group. Another method called *block randomization* can help investigators avoid this potential issue of imbalance in the numbers of people assigned to each study arm by subdividing study participants into blocks of equal size and randomizing the study participants within each block. Each block is associated with a randomization sequence, and this sequence contains an equal number of spots for each study arm (Figure 18.6). However, even if the randomization method used with block randomization was appropriately chosen and carefully carried out, by chance the study arms may not be balanced by prognostic factors. Another method, called *stratified randomization*, is a way to split up or stratify a study sample by one or a few known prognostic factors and randomize study participants within these strata (Figure 18.7). This method preemptively fixes the distribution of these important prognostic factors and between study arms and reduces the probability that by chance the groups will be imbalanced with regard to known prognostic factors.

A rowing event—prognostic balance

A club rowing competition at the Pennsylvania Barge Club was planned to celebrate some of its members' success in winning races at a recent regatta. Although there were eight winners, some were clearly better than others. The planned competition was a 1,000-meter race using two boats with eight oarsmen in each boat. All in all there were the eight winners and eight less accomplished rowers, also with different levels of skills, who were to be allocated to the two boats. Unless the "winners" and the less accomplished rowers were randomly assigned to the boats, there is a potential for a "prognostic imbalance" and an unfair advantage to a boat that may have ended up with more of the better rowers.

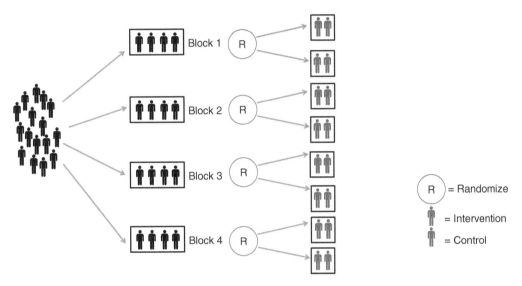

Figure 18.6 Block randomization to reduce an imbalance in the number of study participants in study arms in a randomized controlled trial.

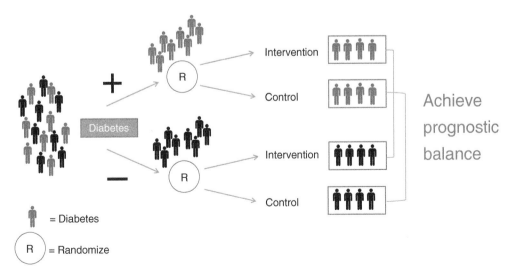

Figure 18.7 Stratified randomization to reduce the chance of imbalance by one or more potential prognostic factors in a randomized controlled trial.

Community service and nonadherence to the protocol

A group of 20 Girl Scouts must complete 40 hours of community service to earn their community service badge. The town has only two options for the girls—they can either pick up trash on the side of the highway or help prepare food at the soup kitchen. It is the middle of winter and everyone would prefer to be in the warm kitchen instead of outside in the cold picking up trash, but both jobs need to be done. The troop leader decides the only fair way to decide which girls will do which task is to randomly allocate them to their assignment. The girls were split evenly, with 10 randomized to pick up trash and 10 randomized to work in the kitchen; 3 of the girls in the trash group were not happy with their assignment and decided to ditch trash day and join the soup kitchen group instead. When the troop leader found out what the girls did they were very upset and had three options when it came time to fill out these 3 girls' community service forms so they could get credit for the hours they worked:

- Option 1: They could ignore the fact that the three girls switched their task from garbage duty to kitchen duty and write on their form that they picked up trash and give them credit for their five hours of service (intention-to-treat analysis)
- Option 2: They could write on their form that they worked in the kitchen and give them credit for their five hours of service (as-treated analysis)
- Option 3: They could refuse to fill out their form, and the girls will get no credit for the five hours they served (naïve per-protocol analysis)

Selected readings

Alshurafa M, Briel M, Akl EA, et al. Inconsistent definitions for intention-to-treat in relation to missing outcome data: systematic review of the methods literature. *Plos One.* 2012;7(11):e49163.

Brignardello-Petersen R, Carrasco-Labra A, Glick M, Guyatt GH, Azarpazhooh A. A practical approach to evidence-based dentistry: III: how to appraise and use an article about therapy. *J Am Dent Assoc.* 2015;146(1):42–49.e1.

Carrasco-Labra A, Brignardello-Petersen R, Azarpazhooh A, Glick M, Guyatt GH. A practical approach to evidence-based dentistry: X: How to avoid being misled by clinical studies' results in dentistry. *J Am Dent Assoc.* 2015;146(12):919–924.

Chalmers I. Comparing like with like: some historical milestones in the evolution of methods to create unbiased comparison groups in therapeutic experiments. *Int J Epidemiol.* 2001;30(5):1156–1164.

Evaniew N, Carrasco-Labra A, Devereaux PJ, et al. How to use a randomized clinical trial addressing a surgical procedure: users' guide to the medical literature. *JAMA Surg.* 2016;151(7):657–662.

Kahale LA, Guyatt GH, Agoritsas T, et al. A guidance was developed to identify participants with missing outcome data in randomized controlled trials. *J Clin Epidemiol.* 2019;115:55–63.

Milojevic M, Nikolic A, Jüni P, Head SJ. A statistical primer on subgroup analyses. *Interact Cardiovasc Thorac Surg.* 2020;30(6):839–845.

Mulla SM, Scott IA, Jackevicius CA, You JJ, Guyatt GH. How to use a noninferiority trial: users' guides to the medical literature. *JAMA.* 2012;308(24):2605–2611.

Schulz KF, Grimes DA. Allocation concealment in randomised trials: defending against deciphering. *Lancet.* 2002;359(9306):614–618.

Sedgwick P. Bias in experimental study designs: randomised controlled trials with parallel groups. *BMJ.* 2015;351:h3869.

19

Understanding and interpreting meta-analyses

Meta-analysis is a statistical technique that synthesizes and combines the results from two or more studies to assess the dispersion of *effects*, distinguish between real and spurious dispersions, and provide a summary effect of all included studies. The result from a meta-analysis is called a *pooled, summary, combined*, or *overall effect estimate*. For simplicity, we refer to it as a pooled estimate herein. Meta-analysis can be conceptualized as a weighted average summary of the results from multiple studies, where each study contributes (provides a different "weight") to the final pooled estimate.

Meta-analyses are robust in the sense that they can combine the results from many study designs (i.e., *randomized control trials* (RCTs), *observational studies*, diagnostic test accuracy studies) (Chapters 15, 16, 17, and 18). Accordingly, meta-analyses can combine relative measures of associate (e.g., *relative risks* (RR), *odds ratios* (OR), *hazard ratios* (HR)), absolute measures of association (e.g., *mean differences* (MD), *standardized mean differences* (SMD), *risk differences* (RD)), and diagnostic test accuracy measures (e.g., *sensitivity*, *specificity*, and diagnostic odds ratios) (Chapters 2, 8, and 9). For example, *continuous outcomes*, like pain intensity, may be measured with visual analog scales ranging from 0 to 10, from 0 to 5, or from 1 to 10. To obtain a single pooled estimate across studies using different scales measuring the same *construct*, scores from these scales can be *standardized* and pooled using a measure of association called the SMD.

The value of meta-analysis

A 67-year-old female saw a television commercial from a company that manufactures vitamin D supplements. The ad recommended that older adults take vitamin D supplements to prevent bone fractures as they age. This patient asked their physician whether it would be beneficial to start taking vitamin D. The physician searched the scientific literature for studies on this topic and found eight RCTs comparing vitamin D supplements with placebo pills and that measured the outcome of bone fracture. The RCTs' *sample* size varied across the eight studies—five found that vitamin D supplements reduced the risk of fractures, but the magnitude of this reduction was large in some studies (80% or RR = 0.20) and much lower in others (10% or RR = 0.90) (Chapter 2). The other three studies suggested that there may be no difference in fractures among those who took vitamin D supplements and those allocated to placebo pills. What should the physician recommend to their patient in the face of the seemingly conflicting results from these eight studies? A meta-analysis summarizing the results of the eight studies would offer just one pooled estimate for the physician to consider when making a recommendation to the patient. Additionally, the physician would be

Statistics for Dental Clinicians, First Edition. Michael Glick, Alonso Carrasco-Labra, and Olivia Urquhart.
© 2024 John Wiley & Sons, Inc. Published 2024 by John Wiley & Sons, Inc.

equipped with a more precise estimate (Chapter 6) than any study alone could have produced. Last, the physician may also be able to find an explanation for the *between-study variance*, a concept called *heterogeneity* (more on this later).

Meta-analyses are usually conducted within a *systematic review* framework. A systematic review is a type of secondary research in which a focused research question drives the search, selection, appraisal, and synthesis of primary studies from the research literature. Studies matching the research question are selected in a stepwise approach, and the data from each study are extracted following standard methodology. If the selected primary studies are similar enough in regard to populations of interest, *interventions/exposures*, comparisons, and outcomes measured, their data can be pooled in a meta-analysis. Systematic reviews are an essential component of *clinical practice guideline* development, so meta-analyses offer a powerful tool for informing clinical decision making at the highest level.

Pairwise meta-analysis

"Pairwise," as the name suggests, refers to the comparison of two groups to yield a pooled treatment effect estimate for the comparison of an outcome between two groups: an active intervention/exposure and another active intervention/exposure, or *placebo*/no exposure. (An "active intervention" is one that is responsible for producing an effect). A comparison could be between two active interventions, for instance, 5% sodium fluoride varnish compared to 1.23% acidulated phosphate fluoride gel for the prevention of caries in children, or an active intervention such as oral analgesics compared to a placebo or no treatment for the management of a toothache.

To derive a pooled *treatment effect* estimate in a *pairwise meta-analysis*, investigators need to compute two components: (1) a treatment effect estimate (e.g., OR, RR, MD) for each primary study and (2) a *weighted* contribution for each primary study. With these two components in hand, a weighted average (i.e., pooled treatment effect estimate) can be calculated. The estimated pooled treatment effect is the quotient of the sum of the product of the treatment effect and the weight from each study, and the sum of the weights for all studies (Appendix 1, Formula 19.1). Studies with larger weights are more influential than those with smaller weights when deriving the pooled treatment effect estimate.

Pairwise meta-analyses can be carried out under two statistical frameworks: *fixed effect meta-analyses* or *random effects meta-analyses*. The choice of framework depends on whether the studies are estimating the same or different effects.

Fixed effect meta-analysis

Consider a hypothetical example of four RCTs comparing the effect of using antibiotics with not using antibiotics and that measured the outcome surgical site infection after third molar extractions in male patients. The four studies were conducted at the same U.S. university hospital. Any differences in the effect on this outcome between these RCTs conducted in the same setting and whose samples were drawn from the same underlying population can be attributed to *within-study variance* (e.g., *random error*) (Chapters 1 and 13). A pooled effect using a fixed effect analysis is based on an underlying assumption that the true effect from all included studies is the same. A fixed effect (also referred to as a common effect or equal effect) meta-analysis allows for the estimation of a pooled effect estimate and a *confidence interval*, where the weight of each primary study contributes to the pooled estimate based solely on the random error.

Random effects meta-analysis

In a second hypothetical scenario, another set of four RCTs answering the same research question presented above are identified from the scientific literature. This time, however, two studies were conducted in Finland, one in Japan, and one in Costa Rica. The surgeons executing the third molar extractions in males in the Finnish studies all performed partial Newman flaps and all were asymptomatic. Males in the Japanese studies received modified Newman flaps and all remained symptomatic. The males participating in the Costa Rican trial had a mixture of Newman and partial Newman flaps and were asymptomatic. The treatment effects in each population from which the study samples were drawn can be expected to be different across the studies. On top of the expected random error, the populations themselves could be different. It is to be expected that there may be variability in the treatment effect between the studies and that the studies are estimating different but related treatment effects. Meta-analysis could still be an appropriate technique to combine the results of these studies; however, instead of accounting for just one type of error (random error), random effects meta-analyses account for an additional type of variability—between-study variability, also called heterogeneity. Because two types of variability are accounted for in a random effects model versus only one type in a fixed effect model, the corresponding confidence intervals tend to be wider under the random effects framework. In other words, estimates from random effects meta-analyses tend to be more conservative. However, when no between-study variability is detected, the fixed and random effects models will result in the same pooled estimate.

Weight of each study in a meta-analysis

The weight corresponds to how much a given study influences or contributes to the pooled effect estimate. Because larger studies have more participants, resulting in smaller *variances* (small standard error) and more narrow confidence intervals compared with smaller studies (larger standard error), they are favored in meta-analyses and are thus given greater weight (Chapter 4). There are different ways to calculate weights depending on whether a fixed effect or a random effects framework is used. One of the most common methods, the *generic inverse-variance method*, can be implemented under both frameworks. As the name implies, the weight is derived by taking the inverse of the variance in each study. Under a fixed effect framework, there is only one type of variance (*within-study variance*), which is depicted by the squared standard error of the effect estimate from each study (Appendix 1, Formula 19.2).

Under a random effects framework, the inverse-variance method uses the same weighting approach as the fixed effect, with one difference. The between-study variance is incorporated in the weight as the inverse of the sum of the squared standard error (within-study variance) and the *between-study variance* (heterogeneity) (often referred to as the square of the Greek letter τ (tau)—τ^2) (Appendix 1, Formula 19.3). Under a random effects framework, smaller studies are assigned larger weights than they would be assigned under a fixed effects framework (Figure 19.1).

Forest plots

A *forest plot* is a graphical representation of the results of a meta-analysis (Figures 19.2 and 19.3). There are many variations of how study data can be displayed in a forest plot depending on the software used, but the main components are all the same. The included studies contributing to the

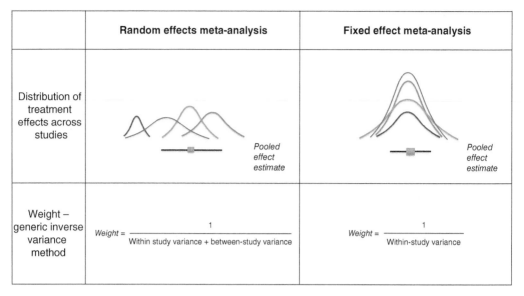

Figure 19.1 Comparison of fixed effect and random effects meta-analysis. The colored curves depict distributions from different samples. The green square represents the point estimate and the horizontal black line depicts the width of the confidence interval.

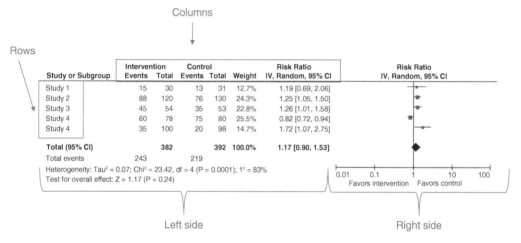

Figure 19.2 Forest plot depicting a meta-analysis of binary data. IV: inverse variance; CI: confidence interval; random: random effects model; df: degree of freedom.

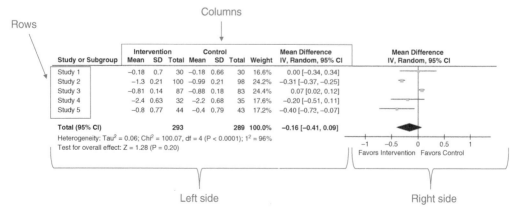

Figure 19.3 Forest plot depicting a meta-analysis of continuous data. IV: inverse variance; SD: standard deviation; CI: confidence interval; random: random effects model; df: degree of freedom.

meta-analysis are listed in the rows. On the left-hand side, every study is represented, often using each author's last name and the year each study was conducted. For *binary outcomes* (Figure 19.2), the number of *events* and total sample size contributing to the analysis are listed for each treatment/ exposure (if available). Analogously, per-study-arm *means*, *standard deviations*, and sample sizes for continuous outcomes are displayed (Figure 19.3). The weight of each study is listed as a column corresponding with each study, with the model type (random effects or fixed effect) and method used to calculate the weights (e.g., inverse-variance (Appendix 1, formulas 19.2 and 19.3), *Mantel–Haenszel*) depicted on the plot. On the right-hand side, the point estimates for the effect of each study are graphically depicted as squares (or some other shape), with the size of the square representing the weight of the study. The width of the corresponding confidence intervals for these estimates are represented by a horizontal line intersecting the square shape. The squares are also placed along the horizontal line according to where the point estimate of the study falls in relation to the no-effect line. These squares and horizontal lines are plotted against an x-axis at the bottom of the plot, with a vertical line, or no-effect line, bisecting the axis. This line divides results from each study according to favoring versus not favoring an intervention or a control. The no-effect line is plotted at 1.0 for relative measures and 0.0 for absolute measures of association (Chapter 2). At the bottom of the plot, the meta-analysis result (pooled estimate) is illustrated with a diamond, whose width corresponds to its confidence interval and its location according to its relationship with the no-effect line. The forest plot figure also contains results of the overall effects test, heterogeneity, and subgroup analysis, if applicable.

Heterogeneity

Do the studies contributing to the meta-analysis tell a similar story? If not, they are deemed to be heterogeneous. There are several explanations for why study results may be different:

1) The clinical characteristics of the studies, such as the participants or the population (e.g., setting, disease severity, age), intervention (e.g., treatment dose, vehicle of administration), and outcomes (e.g., definitions and measures), may differ. On one hand, pooling more broadly by including a more diverse set of components of the research question may increase the generalizability or applicability of the results. On the other hand, the inclusion of a group of studies that are too diverse in the components of the research question may prevent the conduct of a meta-analysis, as the components could be too different.

2) There may be methodological diversity in the studies' design (e.g., factorial vs. cluster design), analysis (e.g., intention-to-treat, per-protocol analysis, or confounders adjusted for), or randomization method (cluster randomized controlled trial vs. randomized block design) (Chapter 18).

3) Statistical heterogeneity or variation in treatment effects will happen by chance. Statistical heterogeneity is the quantifiable aspect of clinical and methodological heterogeneity and tells us if there is more variation than we would expect by chance alone. The more statistical heterogeneity, the lower the certainty in the pooled effect estimate.

Heterogeneity can interfere with the goal of estimating an *unbiased* pooled effect estimate (effect estimate that is close to the true population *parameter*).

Investigators can address heterogeneity in several ways (Table 19.1):

1) Modeling. Heterogeneity can be incorporated into the meta-analysis under a random effects model by estimating the between-study variance, often denoted as τ^2 (tau squared). The practical implication is that the larger the value of τ^2 the wider the confidence interval around the effect estimate. A fixed effect model will ignore the between-study variance. In a random effects

Table 19.1 Strategies used in meta-analysis to address heterogeneity.

Strategy	Implications for strategies
Modeling	Fixed effect model: heterogeneity is ignored Random effects model: heterogeneity is incorporated
Statistical testing (Cochran Q test)	p-value ≥ 0.10 = fail to reject the null hypothesis of no heterogeneity p-value < 0.10 = reject the null hypothesis of no heterogeneity
Quantifying (I^2 statistic)	$I^2 < 25\%$ = low levels of heterogeneity $25\% \leq I^2 \leq 50\%$ = moderate levels of heterogeneity $I^2 > 50\%$ = high levels of heterogeneity
Visualizing (forest plot)	Point estimate alignment: • Non-alignment of point estimates with the pooled estimate = heterogeneity • Alignment of point estimates with the pooled estimate = no heterogeneity Confidence interval overlapping: • No overlap of confidence intervals = heterogeneity • Overlap of confidence intervals = no heterogeneity
Explaining	*Subgroup analysis: test for subgroup differences* p-value for difference in subgroups ≥ 0.05 = fail to reject the null hypothesis of no difference in the effect between subgroups. p-value for difference in subgroups < 0.05 = reject the null hypothesis of no difference in the effect between subgroups. *Meta-regression: estimate and hypothesis test for regression coefficient* Continuous independent variable = the change in the pooled treatment effect when the independent variable changes by one unit Categorical independent variable = the difference in the pooled treatment effect between one level of a subgroup and another level of the subgroup (a reference group). p-value of regression coefficient ≥ 0.05 = fail to reject null hypothesis that there is no difference in effect estimates according to values or levels of a subgroup. p-value of regression coefficient < 0.05 = reject the null hypothesis that there is no difference in effect estimates according to values or levels of a subgroup.

model, if the value for between-study variance is zero, the pooled estimate and confidence interval will be the same between the two models.

2) Statistical testing. Another way to address heterogeneity is by testing for it statistically with *Cochran's Q test*. As expected from hypothesis-testing approaches, this test conveys whether heterogeneity is present or absent. This test is often underpowered to find between-study differences, which warrants the use of a larger level of significance for the test (0.10 instead of the typical 0.05).

3) Quantifying. Heterogeneity can be quantified with a statistic called I^2. The value spans from 0% to 100% and conveys how much variability in the effects across studies can be explained by heterogeneity. Roughly, values lower than 25% can be interpreted as low heterogeneity, between 25% and 50% as moderate, and over 50% as high. This value should be interpreted cautiously when data are sparse.

4) Visualizing. If studies are conducted in a similar fashion, using the same methodology, identical or similar populations, comparable interventions, and so forth, we would not expect large differences in point estimates or confidence intervals between the individual study results. If the point estimates and confidence intervals in a forest plot are generally aligned, the study results may be homogeneous. If they are not generally aligned, there might be some level of

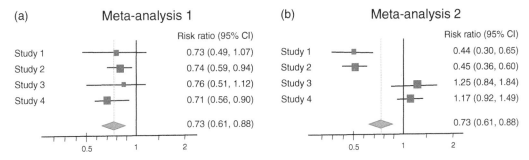

Figure 19.4 Visual inspection of a forest plot to detect heterogeneity in a meta-analysis. (a) No visual evidence of heterogeneity. There is overlap in the point estimates and confidence intervals across studies and all confidence intervals intersect the pooled estimate. (b) Visual evidence of heterogeneity. There is no overlap in the confidence intervals between studies 1 and 2 compared to 3 and 4, and none of the studies contain the point estimate for the pooled result. CI: confidence interval.

heterogeneity. Since statistical tests for heterogeneity are underpowered when the number of included studies is small, an inspection of the forest plot is a key step in ensuring the results of those tests are not spurious (Figure 19.4).

5) Explaining. The results of a group of studies comparing all types of corticosteroids to placebo for a pain relief outcome six hours post-surgery are meta-analyzed. Some studies administered the corticosteroid intramuscularly, some orally, and the rest submucosally. It is hypothesized that submucosal administration will be better at relieving pain compared to the other two modes. A *subgroup analysis* is a way to test the hypothesis that the estimate of effect differs depending on the mode of administration of the corticosteroid. Subgroup analysis in the context of a meta-analysis is a special case of effect modification (Chapter 12). The hypotheses for conducting subgroup analysis should be prespecified and justified based on clinical, biological, or methodological factors.

Another way to investigate subgroup differences is through a *meta-regression*. Subgroup analysis allows for the separation of studies into groups based on some categorical study-level variable, like the mode of administration of a corticosteroid. There may be continuous study-level variables that can help to explain differences in effect estimates across studies; meta-regression helps with this purpose (Chapter 11). In a meta-regression, multiple explanatory variables can be included in the model to predict an outcome variable. Unfortunately, from a practical perspective, meta-regression often has low *power* to detect relationships, as many meta-analyses contain few studies. Rough guidance suggests that there should be at least 10 studies in a meta-analysis for every covariate included in a meta-regression model.

Network meta-analysis

Traditional pairwise meta-analyses are useful for informing the effect of a therapeutic or preventive strategy compared with another strategy, standard of care, or placebo. In clinical practice, however, a variety of therapeutic and preventive options (more than two) may be considered for a single patient. For example, which of corticosteroids, remdesivir, molnupiravir, or hydroxychloroquine is most effective in reducing the length of hospital stay due to COVID-19?[1] Multiple pairwise meta-analyses

1 Siemieniuk RA, Bartoszko JJ, Zeraatkar D, et al. Drug treatments for COVID-19: living systematic review and network meta-analysis [published correction appears in *BMJ*. 2021 Apr 13;373:n967]. *BMJ*. 2020 Jul 30;370:m2980. doi:10.1136/bmj.m2980.

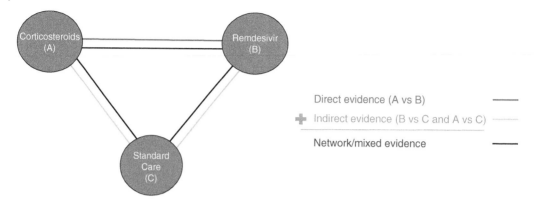

Figure 19.5 Types of evidence that can inform a network meta-analysis.

can answer this question. *Network meta-analysis* is a pairwise meta-analysis derivative that allows for the comparison of three or more interventions simultaneously. This approach combines data for comparisons that have been compared in studies (i.e., *direct effect estimate*) with data for comparisons that have not been compared directly (i.e., *indirect effect estimate*), resulting in a pooled *network* or *mixed treatment effect estimate* (Figure 19.5). Most of the time, this pooled network estimate will be more precise than either the direct or indirect effect estimates alone. Additionally, if two therapeutic interventions have never been compared before in a primary study, network meta-analysis allows one to determine indirect estimates and provide evidence of such a comparative effect.

Sensitivity analysis

Many methodological decisions are made when compiling a dataset that is suitable for meta-analysis. Choosing studies to include in a meta-analysis, classifying the study interventions, and extracting outcome data are just a few decisions researchers face along the way. For instance, in a meta-analysis with mean differences as the *measure of association* (Chapter 2), some of the studies may not report standard deviations and researchers may choose to borrow a known standard deviation from another study included in the same meta-analysis. To check if the meta-analysis result is robust to this arbitrary borrow decision, a *sensitivity analysis* can be conducted. In this approach, first, the meta-analysis is conducted using all the studies, including the one with the borrowed standard deviation, and an effect estimate is obtained. Second, the analysis is conducted again, but this time the study with a borrowed standard deviation is removed from the dataset and an effect estimate is calculated. The pooled point estimate and confidence intervals from the first analysis are compared to those obtained from the second analysis to see if the conclusions differ. If the first and second estimates are similar, researchers can be confident that their results are robust to the borrowing decision. If they differ, there is a possibility that this arbitrary decision and not data from the primary studies biased the conclusions from the meta-analysis.

Certainty of the evidence

The results of meta-analyses conducted in the context of a systematic review should not be taken at face value. After conducting a meta-analysis, it is important to explore possible reasons to question the extent to which the pooled effect estimate is a reflection of the true effect in the population of interest. Many tools for assessing the certainty or quality of the evidence exist. The Grading of Recommendations Assessment, Development and Evaluation (GRADE) approach is one such pervasive tool. In GRADE, the certainty of the evidence rating is determined after exploring five domains that can rate down the certainty: risk of bias, inconsistency (or heterogeneity), publication bias, indirectness, and imprecision; and three domains that can rate up the certainty: large magnitude of effect, dose-response gradient, and when residual confounding is likely to decrease rather than increase the magnitude of the observed effect.

A few additional notes

- Many methods are available to estimate between-study variance or τ^2 (e.g., DerSimonian and Laird, maximum likelihood, etc.), with some more advantageous than others under certain conditions.
- Under both fixed effect and random effects frameworks, there are methods in addition to the *generic inverse-variance method* to calculate weights for each study. Some of the most common include the Mantel–Haenszel and *Peto's methods*. The Mantel–Haenszel method performs well when data are sparse, meaning when either the event rates or sample sizes of the studies are small. Peto can be used only to pool ORs, in contrast to the other two methods, which have more versatility. Peto tends to perform well when the OR is close to 1 and the sample size in the arms of the study are balanced but less well when the magnitude of the treatment effect is large.
- We can test for the presence or absence of heterogeneity with Cochran's Q test. The null hypothesis for this test is $\tau^2 = 0$, or that all studies are estimating the same effect, and the alternative hypothesis is $\tau^2 > 0$, or that at least one study has an effect different from the pooled effect estimate. Statistically nonsignificant p-values indicate that the null hypothesis of no heterogeneity (i.e., homogeneity) cannot be rejected. When the data are sparse, which is often the case when conducting meta-analyses, this test has low power, so statistically nonsignificant p-values are not necessarily a definitive indication that no heterogeneity exists.
- Subgroup analyses are typically underpowered, and failure to detect a difference in treatment effects between subgroups does not mean one may not exist.
- Meta-regression is a derivative of linear regression, where the regression coefficients for a continuous covariate correspond to the percentage increase in the outcome variable for a one-unit change in the explanatory variable. For categorical variables, the regression coefficient represents the difference between one level (the reference group) and other levels of the categorical variable.
- Measures obtained from diagnostic test accuracy studies can also be meta-analyzed. When the measure is a diagnostic odds ratio (Chapter 9), the standard fixed effect and random effects meta-analysis models will produce valid results. Since measures like sensitivity and specificity are correlated (Chapter 10), different meta-analytic approaches (*bivariate random effects model* or a *hierarchical summary receiver operating curve* model) can account for this *correlation*.

Application of a weighted average to average salaries among females and males

Only looking and comparing individual studies without an estimated weighted average may not correctly represent a pooled estimate. For example: There are 90 male physicians making an average annual salary of $100,000 and 40 female physicians earning an average of $110,000.

There are 10 male nurses making an average annual salary of $40,000 and 60 female nurses earning an average of $44,000.

Thus, in each profession females have higher average salaries. However, the average salary of all males is $94,000, while that of all females is $70,400. The average female salary is lower than that of males.

Even though females earn more money on average than males within each profession, many more (90 in total) male physicians contribute to a higher salary compared to female physicians (40 in total) (i.e., males contribute a larger weight) and very few male nurses (10 in total) contribute to a lower salary compared to female nurses (60 in total) (i.e., males contribute a smaller weight); therefore, the overall average salary is higher for males than for females.

Profession	Males		Females		Higher salary?
	Number	Average salary	Number	Average salary	
physician	90	$100,000.00	40	**$110,000.00**	Women
Nurse	10	$40,000.00	60	**$44,000.00**	Women
Total	100	**$94,000.00**	100	$70,400.00	Men

Selected readings

Cordero CP, Dans AL. Key concepts in clinical epidemiology: detecting and dealing with heterogeneity in meta-analyses. *J Clin Epidemiol.* 2021;130:149–151.

Higgins JPT, Thomas J, Chandler J, Cumpston M, Li T, Page MJ, Welch VA, eds. *Cochrane Handbook for Systematic Reviews of Interventions*, version 6.3 (updated February 2022). Cochrane; 2022. Available from www.training.cochrane.org/handbook.

Rochwerg B, Brignardello-Petersen R, Guyatt G. Network meta-analysis in health care decision making. *Med J Aust.* 2018;209(4):151–154.

Sedgwick P. How to read a forest plot in a meta-analysis. *BMJ.* 2015;351:h4028.

Sedgwick P. Meta-analyses: heterogeneity and subgroup analysis. *BMJ.* 2013;346:f4040.

Sedgwick P. Meta-analyses: What is heterogeneity? *BMJ.* 2015;350:h1435.

Sun X, Ioannidis JP, Agoritsas T, Alba AC, Guyatt G. How to use a subgroup analysis: users' guide to the medical literature. *JAMA.* 2014;311(4):405–411.

20

Understanding and interpreting statistical and clinical significance

The primary purpose of clinical research is to identify *risk* and *prognostic factors*, diagnostic tests, and preventive and therapeutic *interventions* that help maintain the health of individuals, recover the health of those who are sick, or mitigate the impact of living with a disease. Clinical research is, in essence, applicable to clinical practice and policy. The scientific and clinical community determines that a new health intervention should be adopted following a long process that connects basic, translational, and applied research. Throughout that process, the safety and effectiveness profile of the new intervention is determined.

To distinguish between anomalies and true results, the scientific community has focused on *hypothesis testing* and *p-values* (Chapter 5). These methods focus primarily on the premise that a study treatment makes no difference in an *outcome* of interest (*null hypothesis*). The p-value reflects the compatibility or similarity between the data collected by the investigators and a prespecified model (e.g., t-statistic, chi-squared statistic) by providing a measure of the *probability* that the preselected test statistic would have been at least as large as the value observed in the study, under several assumptions. These assumptions include that the study was conducted free from *bias* and *confounding*, outcomes were measured using reliable and valid methods, the *sample* was a representative group of the population to which the results will be applied, the null hypothesis is true, and more. P-values are frequently used as means to determine whether a health intervention provides a health benefit. Unfortunately, this information cannot be derived from p-values. A more appropriate approach would be to provide an assessment of the level of uncertainty regarding the size of an effect. One fundamental flaw of using hypothesis testing methods to determine the clinical relevance of a study's result is the tendency to equate *statistical significance* with practical importance or *clinical significance*. Since p-values cannot help to determine the certainty around the size of an effect, other alternatives have emerged that can provide patients and clinicians with that necessary information. A consensus has emerged to focus on estimation methods with the presentation of *confidence intervals* (CIs) (Chapter 6). Because they provide a range of plausible results in the same units as the outcome measure of interest, CIs represent progress toward making research findings more easily and broadly accessible and applicable. Having a range of plausible results that may contain the true effect allows users of research findings to understand the practical implications of the upper and lower boundaries of the CI.

The apparent solution of using CIs to determine the practical value of a health intervention comes with important assumptions and challenges. For example, when presented with a CI, one cannot know whether that CI contains the true size of the effect of interest; however, users and researchers always proceed as if such an interval does contain the true value (Chapter 6). Moving

Statistics for Dental Clinicians, First Edition. Michael Glick, Alonso Carrasco-Labra, and Olivia Urquhart.
© 2024 John Wiley & Sons, Inc. Published 2024 by John Wiley & Sons, Inc.

from hypothesis testing to estimation methods using CIs may solve the problem of interpreting study results in an oversimplistic, binary manner—an intervention shows or does not show statistically significant differences compared to a control. However, it brings challenges in interpreting the interval and its practical implications, especially the range of values contained within the CI that patients, clinicians, and society would consider meaningful. Thus, instead of obtaining a yes/no answer, estimation methods allow for the determination of the extent to which the size of an effect is negligible or trivial (and is not worthy of our attention), small but important, moderate, or large. However, the issue of defining a threshold to evaluate the extent to which a *treatment effect* can be judged as unimportant or important remains.

A *minimal important difference* addresses the challenges in interpreting outcome measures, particularly the need to establish a threshold to distinguish an unimportant (or trivial) from a small but important effect. This measure represents the smallest change—improvement or deterioration—in an outcome of interest, either beneficial or harmful, that people would perceive as important. The definition of these thresholds of clinical significance should be informed by evidence, defined on a case-by-case basis, and identified using several criteria, including the frequency and severity of the outcome of interest, the lack of other treatment availability, the costs and burden or level of invasiveness of the intervention, and the relative importance of the outcome of interest in the context of other outcomes expected from the intervention. These criteria move the threshold up or down accordingly.

Figure 20.1 shows a *forest plot* (Chapter 19), including a series of seven hypothetical *randomized controlled trials* (Chapter 18) conducted to determine the effect of dental sealants compared with not using dental sealants on the *incidence* of caries lesions. The blue squares are the studies' point estimates, the squares' size represents the study *precision (standard error)* (Chapter 4), and the thin horizontal line overlapping the squares shows their 95% CIs (Chapter 6). Determining statistical and clinical significance requires prespecification of thresholds. The threshold for determining statistical significance has been set up by convention within the research community at 5% (level of

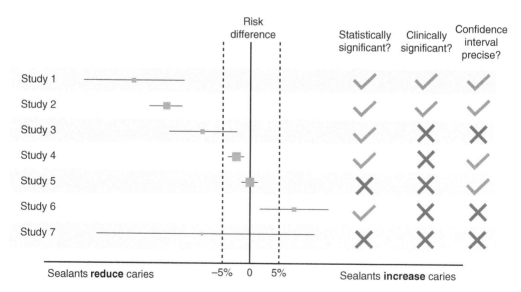

Figure 20.1 Statistical significance, clinical significance, and confidence interval precision for a hypothetical series of seven studies reporting on the absolute effect of dental sealants compared with no sealants use on caries lesion incidence.

significance of 0.05). The solid vertical line is the line of no effect, which for a *risk difference* is zero (Chapter 2). A CI crossing this threshold includes the possibility of no difference between receiving and not receiving a dental sealant. The practical implication is that such a CI will show results that are not statistically significant. The threshold to determine clinical significance is rarely reported in studies published in the research literature. In this example, the dotted lines to the right and the left of the no-effect line are the minimal important difference thresholds to claim that dental sealants offer a reduction (left side) or increase (right side) in the incidence of caries lesions that is, at least, small but important from a clinical point of view. In this example, the minimal important difference is set at a 5% reduction or increase in the incidence of caries lesions. The CI for study 1 lies to the left of the clinical and statistical significant thresholds, which means that the results are both clinically and statistically significant (dotted line). The upper and lower boundaries of the 95% CI suggest that dental sealants are effective in reducing the incidence of caries lesions. Study 2 shows similar results to study 1, with analogous practical implications, although the 95% CI is more precise.

The CI of study 3 crosses the threshold for clinical significance (dotted line) but does not cross the threshold for statistical significance. This means that these results may not be clinically significant but are statistically significant. The upper and lower boundaries of the 95% CI include the possibility of an effect larger and smaller than the clinically significant threshold. This discrepancy prevents us from ascertaining whether sealants truly have an important effect, which indicates that the CI for study 3 is imprecise. Notice that statistically significant study results reflected in a 95% CI may still have issues of imprecision.

The 95% CI for study 4 lies between the clinical and statistical significance thresholds and does not cross either of them, indicating that there may not be issues of imprecision. Its upper and lower boundaries suggest that although the difference in caries incidence between using and not using dental sealants may be statistically significant, it is certainly not clinically significant (the entire 95% CI lying to the right of the clinical significance threshold). In other words, based on the results of study 4, if any benefit from dental sealants is expected, it is negligible. The 95% CI for study 4 is precise as it does not cross the clinical significance thresholds.

The 95% CI for study 5 lies right on top of the statistical significance threshold, suggesting that the difference observed may not be statistically significant. Its upper and lower boundaries suggest that dental sealants versus not using dental sealants may result in a negligible benefit (area to the right (−5% to 0) of the clinical significance thresholds) or negligible harm (area to the left (5% to 0) of the clinical significance thresholds). This indicates that there may not be a clinically significant difference between using and not using dental sealants. In other words, based on study 5's findings, dental sealants do not have an effect on the incidence of caries lesions. The 95% CI does not cross the clinical significance threshold, suggesting that these results do not have issues of impression. Notice that from a statistical standpoint, the 95% CIs of studies 4 and 5 show dissimilar conclusions—study 4 is statistically significant, study 5 is not. However, the implications for practice are the same for both: sealants would not help to reduce the incidence of caries lesions enough to be clinically helpful.

Study 6 has implications for clinical and statistical significance that are similar to those of study 3 (results that are statistically but not clinically significant and an imprecise 95% CI). However, the practical implications associated with these results warrant not using sealants in clinical practice, as both boundaries of the 95% CI reside on the side of harm, suggesting that sealants may increase the incidence of caries lesions.

Study 7 has the least precise of all 95% CIs in the figure and is expected to have the largest standard error (Chapter 4). This imprecision is verified in the CI crossing both clinical significance thresholds (−5% and 5%), suggesting a potentially large benefit (left boundary of the CI), no difference (crossing the no-effect line), and possible large harm (right boundary of the CI) when using sealants compared to not using sealants. In addition, this CI crosses the line of no effect, indicating that the results are not statistically significant, and crosses both clinical significant thresholds, indicating that the results may not be clinically significant.

A few additional notes

- Disregard research finding statements claiming clinical significance on the basis of providing evidence only of statistical significance.
- Look for *measures of association* (Chapter 2), interpret the estimate, and make a judgment as to whether the size of the effect reported in the study is negligible, small but important, moderate, or large.
- Beware of research finding statements of equivalence between two interventions (e.g., investigators fail to reject the null hypothesis, so they conclude that either intervention would show a similar treatment effect) based on a lack of statistical significance (Chapter 7).
- Interventions always have desirable and undesirable consequences that should be reported in clinical studies as outcomes of benefit and harm. Remain skeptical when presented with the size of an effect of an intervention for a single outcome as the basis to claim clinical significance or recommend a change in clinical practice. Both benefits and harms should be weighed with one another to properly claim that an intervention provides a net health benefit.

Setting a significant threshold and deciding on a child's allowance

To teach a ten-year-old child how to be responsible with money, two parents discussed giving her a monthly allowance. One parent argued that they have to carefully determine how much money to give her. Too little would make the entire exercise futile as she would not be able to buy anything or would need to save money for too long. Too much and she will be spoiled and likely waste the money. Thus, the allowance should be large enough for the child to cover fixed expenses, such as some snacks at school, and also be able to save money to buy toys or sporting goods. At the same time, the allowance should be small enough to give the child a sense of scarcity and inculcate a need for financial responsibility. The parents sat together and created a budget for the child and determined the exact allowance amount. This amount represents a threshold, and the parents' discussion highlights the different elements that determine how that threshold may move up or down. Thus, the parents determined the smallest amount of money for the allowance that will be important for the child to learn how to be financially responsible. This resembles a minimal important difference.

Selected readings

Brignardello-Petersen R, Carrasco-Labra A, Shah P, Azarpazhooh A. A practitioner's guide to developing critical appraisal skills: what is the difference between clinical and statistical significance? *J Am Dent Assoc.* 2013 Jul;144(7):780–786.

Carrasco-Labra A, Brignardello-Petersen R, Azarpazhooh A, Glick M, Guyatt GH. A practical approach to evidence-based dentistry: X: How to avoid being misled by clinical studies' results in dentistry. *J Am Dent Assoc.* 2015 Dec;146(12):919–924.

Carrasco-Labra A, Devji T, Qasim A, Phillips MR, et al. Minimal important difference estimates for patient-reported outcomes: a systematic survey. *J Clin Epidemiol.* 2021 May;133:61–71.

Greenland S, Senn SJ, Rothman KJ, Carlin JB, Poole C, Goodman SN, Altman DG. Statistical tests, P values, confidence intervals, and power: a guide to misinterpretations. *Eur J Epidemiol.* 2016 Apr;31(4):337–350.

Jaeschke R, Singer J, Guyatt GH. Measurement of health status. Ascertaining the minimal clinically important difference. *Control Clin Trials.* 1989 Dec;10(4):407–415.

Ranganathan P, Pramesh CS, Buyse M. Common pitfalls in statistical analysis: clinical versus statistical significance. *Perspect Clin Res.* 2015 Jul–Sep;6(3):169–170.

Schünemann HJ, Guyatt GH. Commentary—goodbye M©ID! Hello MID, where do you come from? *Health Serv Res.* 2005 Apr;40(2):593–597.

Sedgwick P. Clinical significance versus statistical significance. *BMJ.* 2014; 348:g2130.

Sedgwick P. What is significance? *BMJ.* 2015;350:h3475.

Yaddanapudi LN. The American Statistical Association statement on P-values explained. *J Anaesthesiol Clin Pharmacol.* 2016 Oct–Dec;32(4):421–423.

Appendix 1

Formulas and equations

Notations used in formulas and equations

α—significance level

β—1− power; regression coefficient

ε—residual term

θ—unknown parameter; pooled effect estimate in meta-analyses

κ—Cohen's kappa

μ_i—mean of population i

σ—population standard deviation

$\sigma_{\hat{p}}$—standard deviation of p

$\sigma_{\bar{x}}$—standard deviation of $\bar{x}$

τ^2—between-study variability, random effects meta-analysis

N—number of observations in the population

N_i—number of observations in population i

P—proportion of successes in the population; incidence

P(X)—probability of having an outcome

P($\hat{X}$)—estimate of the population probability for having an outcome

SE_i—standard error of effect estimate for study, i, in a meta-analysis

$SE_{\hat{p}}$—standard error of p

$SE_{\bar{x}}$—standard error of $\bar{x}$

$SE_{\bar{x}_1 - \bar{x}_2}$—standard error of the difference of means

W_i—weight of study i, in a meta-analysis

X_i—a given value, i, for the independent variable

Y_i—treatment effect for study i

a—y-intercept

b—slope of the line

n—number of observations in the sample

n_i—number of observations in sample i

p—proportion of successes in the sample

p_i—proportion of successes in the sample i

$\hat{p}_i$—"p-hat," estimate of a sample proportion for sample i

$\hat{p}$—"p-hat," estimate of pooled sample proportion; mean of a sample proportion

$s_{\hat{p}}$—sample standard deviation of a proportion; sample estimate of $\sigma_{\hat{p}}$

s_{pooled}—a weighted average of standard deviations for two or more groups

$s_{\bar{x}}$—sample standard deviation of a mean; sample estimate of $\sigma_{\bar{x}}$

t—t-statistic

x—value of the independent variable

$\bar{x}$—"x-bar," sample mean; sample estimate of population mean (μ)

$\bar{x}_i$—mean of the sample i; sample estimate of μ_i

y—value of the independent variable

$\hat{y}_i$—(y-hat), estimate of population mean for a given value, i, for the dependent variable

z—z-score for a sample

$z_{\bar{x}}$—z-score for a sample mean

z_{SEM}—z-score for standard error of the mean

Mathematical symbols and notations

Σ—sum of a number of similar terms

$\propto$—proportional to

$\neq$—not equal to

$\approx$—almost equal to

∞—infinity

Statistics for Dental Clinicians, First Edition. Michael Glick, Alonso Carrasco-Labra, and Olivia Urquhart.
© 2024 John Wiley & Sons, Inc. Published 2024 by John Wiley & Sons, Inc.

Chapter 1   What is statistics and why do we need it?

Formula 1.1 Incidence proportion

$$\text{Incidence proportion} = \frac{\sum \text{new positive cases during a specific time period}}{\sum \text{total population without the disease at baseline}}$$

Formula 1.2 Incidence rate

$$\text{Incidence rate} = \frac{\sum \text{new positive cases during a specific time period}}{\sum \text{person} - \text{time at risk}}$$

Formula 1.3 Prevalence

$$\text{Prevalence} = \frac{\sum \text{positive cases at a specific time}}{\sum \text{total population at baseline}}$$

Formula 1.4 Mean of a population

$$\mu_i = \frac{\sum_{i=1}^{N} X_i}{N}$$

Formula 1.5 Mean of a sample

$$\bar{x} = \frac{x_1 + x_2 + \ldots + x_n}{n} = \frac{\sum_{i=1}^{n} X_i}{n}$$

Formula 1.6 Mean of a sample proportion

$$\hat{p} = \frac{\sum_{i=1}^{n} p_i}{n}$$

Formula 1.7 Median

odd number (n) of ordered observations in a set: $\frac{n+1}{2}$ is the place of the median value

even number (n) of ordered observations in a set: $\dfrac{\left(\dfrac{n}{2}\right) + \left(\dfrac{n}{2} + 1\right)}{2}$ is the estimated place of the median value

Chapter 2   Understanding and interpreting measures of association

	Condition present	Condition absent	
Exposure present (exposed)	a	b	a+b
Exposure absent (unexposed)	c	d	c+d
	a+c	b+d	a+b+c+d

Formula 2.1 Absolute risk (AR) (exposed)

$$AR_{exposed} = \frac{a}{a+b}$$

Formula 2.2 Absolute risk (AR) (unexposed)

$$AR_{unexposed} = \frac{c}{c+d}$$

Formula 2.3 Absolute risk difference (ARD)

$$ARD = AR_{exposed} - AR_{unexposed} = \frac{a}{a+b} - \frac{c}{c+d}$$

Formula 2.4 Relative risk (RR) (exposed relative to unexposed)

$$RR = \frac{AR_{exposed}}{AR_{unexposed}} = \frac{\frac{a}{a+b}}{\frac{c}{c+d}}$$

Formula. 2.5 Relative risk difference (RRD)

$$RRD = \left(\frac{AR_{exposed} - AR_{unexposed}}{AR_{unexposed}}\right) \times 100 = \left(\frac{\frac{a}{a+b} - \frac{c}{c+d}}{\frac{c}{c+d}}\right) \times 100 = \left(\frac{\frac{a}{a+b}}{\frac{c}{c+d}} - 1\right) \times 100 = (RR - 1) \times 100$$

Formula 2.6a Odds of condition among exposed individuals

$$Odds_{exposed} = \frac{a}{b}$$

Formula 2.6b Odds of condition among unexposed individuals

$$\text{Odds}_{\text{unexposed}} = \frac{c}{d}$$

Formula 2.7 Odds ratio (OR) for odds of condition among exposed individuals relative to unexposed individuals

$$\text{OR} = \frac{\text{odds of the condition among exposed individuals}}{\text{odds of the condition among unexposed individuals}} = \frac{\dfrac{a}{b}}{\dfrac{c}{d}} = \frac{ad}{bc}$$

Formula 2.8a Odds of being exposed among individuals with the condition

$$\text{Odds}_{\text{condition+}} = \frac{a}{c}$$

Formula 2.8b Odds of being exposed among individuals without the condition

$$\text{Odds}_{\text{condition-}} = \frac{b}{d}$$

Formula 2.9 Odds ratio (OR) for odds of exposure among individuals with the condition relative to individuals without the condition

$$\text{OR} = \frac{\text{odds of exposure among individuals with the condition}}{\text{odds of exposure among individuals without the condition}} = \frac{\dfrac{a}{c}}{\dfrac{b}{d}} = \frac{ad}{bc}$$

Formula 2.10 Converting an odds ratio (OR) to a relative risk (RR) at a different incidence level (P)

$$\text{RR} = \frac{\text{OR}}{1 - P + (P \times \text{OR})}$$

Formula 2.11 Mean difference (MD)

$$\text{MD} = \mu_1 - \mu_2$$

Equation 2.1a Absolute risk (AR) (exposed)

$$\text{AR}_{\text{exposed}} = \frac{650}{650 + 350} = 0.65 = 65\% \qquad \text{(Formula 2.1)}$$

Equation 2.1b Absolute risk (AR) (unexposed)

$$AR_{unexposed} = \frac{150}{150 + 850} = 0.15 = 15\% \qquad \text{(Formula 2.2)}$$

Equation 2.2 Absolute risk difference (ARD)

$$ARD = \frac{650}{650 + 350} - \frac{150}{150 + 850} = 0.65 - 0.15 = 0.50 = 50 \text{ percentage points} \qquad \text{(Formula 2.3)}$$

Equation 2.3a Relative risk (RR) (exposed relative to unexposed)

$$RR = \frac{\dfrac{650}{650 + 350}}{\dfrac{150}{150 + 850}} = 4.33 \qquad \text{(Formula 2.4)}$$

Equation 2.3b Relative risk difference (RRD)

$$RRD = \left(\frac{\dfrac{650}{650 + 350}}{\dfrac{150}{150 + 850}} - 1 \right) \times 100 = 333\% \qquad \text{(Formula 2.5)}$$

Equation 2.4a

$$\text{Odds of developing periodontal disease among smokers} = \frac{650}{350} = 1.86 \qquad \text{(Formula 2.6a)}$$

$$\text{Odds of developing periodontal disease among non} - \text{smokers} = \frac{150}{850} = 0.18 \qquad \text{(Formula 2.6b)}$$

Equation 2.4b

Odds ratio (OR) for odds of periodontal disease among smokers relative to odds of periodontal disease among nonsmokers

$$OR = \frac{650 \times 850}{350 \times 150} = 10.52 \qquad \text{(Formula 2.7)}$$

Equation 2.5a

$$\text{Odds of being a smoker among those with periodontal disease} = \frac{650}{150} = 4.33 \qquad \text{(Formula 2.8a)}$$

$$\text{Odds of being a smoker among those without periodontal disease} = \frac{350}{850} = 0.41 \qquad \text{(Formula 2.8b)}$$

Equation 2.5b Odds ratio (OR) for odds of being a smoker among individuals with periodontal disease relative to odds of being a nonsmoker among individuals without periodontal disease

$$OR = \frac{650 \times 850}{350 \times 150} = 10.52$$

(Formula 2.9)

Equation 2.6 Mean difference (MD)

$$MD = 1.5 \, mm - 3.5 \, mm = -2.0 \, mm$$

Chapter 3 Understanding and interpreting a standard deviation and normal distribution

Formula 3.1a z-score for the difference between a sample mean and the population mean

$$z_{\bar{x}} = \frac{raw\ score - mean}{standard\ deviation} \ or = \frac{x_i - \mu}{\sigma_{\bar{x}}}; z_i = \frac{x_i - \bar{x}}{s_{\bar{x}}}; s_{\bar{x}} \text{ is a good estimation for } \sigma_{\bar{x}} \text{ when n is large } (>30)$$

Formula 3.1b z-score for standard error of the mean (SE)

$$z_{SEM} = \frac{sample\ mean - population\ mean}{standard\ error\ of\ the\ mean} \ or = \frac{\bar{X} - \mu}{SEM}$$

Formula 3.2 Standard deviation—sample mean

$$s_{\bar{x}} = \sqrt{\frac{\sum_{i=1}^{n} (x_i - \bar{x})^2}{n-1}}$$

Formula 3.3 Standard deviation of a sample proportion

$$s_{\hat{p}} = \sqrt{\frac{p(1-p)}{n}}$$

Equation 3.1 Estimating a z-score for 3 mm where the mean is 2.70 mm and the standard deviation is 0.44 mm.

Mean $(\bar{x}) = 2.70$ mm; standard deviation (s) = 0.44 mm

$$z = \frac{3.0 - 2.7}{0.44} = 0.68$$

(Formula 3.1a)

A z-score of 0.68 equals 0.7517 or 75.17% (Appendix 2).

Chapter 4 Understanding and interpreting standard error

The standard deviation of the population (σ), the standard deviation of the sample (σ_x), the standard deviation of the mean itself ($\hat{\sigma}_{\bar{x}}$), (which is the standard error), and the estimator of the standard deviation of the mean ($\hat{\sigma}_{\bar{x}}$), which is the most often calculated quantity, are often used synonymously. The actual standard error of the mean (SEM) is $\hat{\sigma}_{\bar{x}}$ but this notation is seldom used in the biomedical literature.

Formula 4.1 Standard error of the mean (SEM)

$$SE_{\bar{x}} = \frac{s_{\bar{x}}}{\sqrt{n}}$$

Formula 4.2 95% confidence interval (95% CI)

$$\bar{x} \pm z_{\alpha/2}\frac{\sigma_{\bar{x}}}{\sqrt{n}}; \ \bar{x} \pm z_{\alpha/2}\left(SE_{\bar{x}}\right); \ \bar{x} \pm 1.96 \times SE_{\bar{x}}$$

Formula 4.3 Estimating a p-value for differences of means

Step 1. Pooled standard deviation (SD)

$$s_{pooled} = \sqrt{\frac{\left(n_1-1\right)\left(s_{\hat{p}1}\right)^2 + \left(n_2-1\right)\left(s_{\hat{p}2}\right)^2}{n_1+n_2-2}}$$

Step 2. Standard error of the difference of the means

$$SE_{\bar{x}_1-\bar{x}_2} = \left(s_{pooled}\right) x\sqrt{\frac{1}{n_1}+\frac{1}{n_2}}$$

Step 3. Calculate the t-statistic*

$$t = \frac{\bar{x}_1 - \bar{x}_2}{SE_{\bar{x}_1-\bar{x}_2}}$$

Step 4. Look up the P-value for the t-statistic in a t-table*

$$t = \frac{\bar{x}_1 - \bar{x}_2}{SE_{\bar{x}_1-\bar{x}_2}}$$

Equation 4.1 Estimating the SE

$$\text{Group 1: } \frac{8.76}{\sqrt{10}} = 2.77; \text{ Group 2: } \frac{10.05}{\sqrt{10}} = 3.18$$

Equation 4.2 95% confidence interval (95% CI)

$$\text{Group 1} - 122.90 \pm 1.96 \times 2.77 \rightarrow 117.47 \text{ to } 128.33$$

$$\text{Group 2} - 113.80 \pm 1.96 \times 3.18 \rightarrow 107.57 \text{ to } 120.03$$

Equation 4.3 Estimating a p-value for differences of means

$$\text{Step 1. } s_{pooled} = \sqrt{\frac{\left(10-1\right)8.76^2 + \left(10-1\right)10.05^2}{10+10-2}} = 9.42$$

Step 2. $SE_{\bar{x}_1 - \bar{x}_2} = (9.42) \times \sqrt{\dfrac{1}{10} + \dfrac{1}{10}} = 4.22$

Step 3. $t = \dfrac{113.8 - 122.9}{4.22} = 2.16$

Step 4. p-value = 0.04

*For the t-statistic, a t-table instead of a z-table should be used.

Chapter 5   Understanding and interpreting hypothesis testing and p-values

Formula 5.1 Pooled sample proportion

$$\hat{p} = \frac{\text{sum of successes in group 1 and group 2}}{\text{total number of individuals}} = \frac{\hat{p}_1 n_1 + \hat{p}_2 n_2}{n_1 + n_2}$$

Formula 5.2 z-score for the difference in sample proportions

$$z = \frac{\hat{p}_1 - \hat{p}_2}{\sqrt{\hat{p}(1-\hat{p})(\dfrac{1}{n_1} + \dfrac{1}{n_2})}}$$

Equation 5.1 Pooled sample proportion

$$\hat{p} = \frac{\dfrac{62}{95} \times 95 + \dfrac{48}{95} \times 95}{95 + 95} = 0.5789 \qquad \text{(Formula 5.1)}$$

Equation 5.2 z-score for the difference in sample proportions

$$z = \frac{\dfrac{62}{95} - \dfrac{48}{95}}{\sqrt{(0.5789)(1 - 0.5789)(\dfrac{1}{95} + \dfrac{1}{95})}} = 2.06 \qquad \text{(Formula 5.2)}$$

z-score of 2.06 equals a probability of 0.98, and a probability of group 1 being better is p-value = 1 − 0.98 = 0.02; if this was a 2-tailed hypothesis, p-value = 0.04 (Appendix 2).

Equation 5.3

		G_{11}	G_{12}
Mean (mm Hg)	$\bar{x}_{11}, \bar{x}_{12}$	105.0	108.5
Mean difference (mm Hg)	$\bar{x}_{11} - \bar{x}_{12}$ (Formula 2.11)	105.0 − 108.5 = −3.5	
Sample size	n_{11}, n_{12}	15	15
Standard deviation (SD)	s_{11}, s_{12}	12.4	10.8

(Continued)

	G_{11}	G_{12}
Pooled SD	$s_{pooled} = \sqrt{\dfrac{(n_{11}-1)(s_{11})^2 + (n_{12}-1)(s_{12})^2}{n_{11}+n_{12}-2}}$ (Formula 4.3)	$\sqrt{\dfrac{(15-1)(12.4)^2 + (15-1)(10.8)^2}{15+15-2}} = 11.63$
Standard error (SE) of mean difference	$SE_{\bar{x}_1 - \bar{x}_2} = s_{pooled}\sqrt{\dfrac{1}{n_{11}} + \dfrac{1}{n_{12}}}$ (Formula 4.3)	$11.63\sqrt{\dfrac{1}{15} + \dfrac{1}{15}} = 4.25$
Test statistics	$\dfrac{\bar{x}_{11} - \bar{x}_{12}}{SE_{\bar{x}_1 - \bar{x}_2}}$	$\dfrac{105.0 - 108.5}{4.25} = -0.82$
Degree of freedom (df)	$n_{11} + n_{12} - 2$	28
p-value	$t \le -\dfrac{\bar{x}_{11} - \bar{x}_{12}}{SE_{\bar{x}_1 - \bar{x}_2}}$ or $t \ge -\dfrac{\bar{x}_{11} - \bar{x}_{12}}{SE_{\bar{x}_1 - \bar{x}_2}}$	0.417*

* For the t-statistic, a t-table (Appendix 3) instead of a z-table (Appendix 2) should be used.

Equation 5.4

		G_{21}	G_{22}
Mean (mm Hg)	$\bar{x}_{21}, \bar{x}_{22}$	105.0	108.5
Mean difference (mm Hg)	$\bar{x}_{21} - \bar{x}_{22}$	-3.5	
Sample size	n_{21}, n_{22}	15	15
Standard deviation (SD)	s_{21}, s_{22}	3.9	3.8
Pooled SD	$s_{pooled} = \sqrt{\dfrac{(n_{11}-1)(s_{11})^2 + (n_{12}-1)(s_{12})^2}{n_{11}+n_{12}-2}}$	$\sqrt{\dfrac{(15-1)(3.9)^2 + (15-1)(3.8)^2}{15+15-2}} = 3.85$	
Standard error (SE) of mean difference	$SE_{\bar{x}_1 - \bar{x}_2} = s\sqrt{\dfrac{1}{n_{21}} + \dfrac{1}{n_{22}}}$ (Formula 4.3)	$3.85\sqrt{\dfrac{1}{15} + \dfrac{1}{15}} = 1.41$	
Test statistics	$\dfrac{\bar{x}_{21} - \bar{x}_{22}}{SE_{\bar{x}_1 - \bar{x}_2}}$	$\dfrac{105.0 - 108.5}{1.41} = -2.49$	
Degree of freedom (df)	$n_{21} + n_{22} - 2$	28	
p-value	$t \le -\dfrac{\bar{x}_{21} - \bar{x}_{22}}{SE}$ or $t \ge -\dfrac{\bar{x}_{21} - \bar{x}_{22}}{SE}$	0.019*	

* For the t-statistic, a t-table instead of a z-table should be used.

Chapter 6 Understanding and interpreting a confidence interval

Formula 6.1a z-score

$$z_{\alpha/2} \text{ (Appendix 2)}$$

Formula 6.1b Margin of error—continuous variables

$$\pm\, z_{\alpha/2}\text{SE} = \pm\, z_{\alpha/2}\frac{\sigma}{\sqrt{n}} \text{ if } \sigma_{\bar{x}} \text{ is unknown, replace z for t, and } \mu \text{ with } \bar{x}$$

Formula 6.1c Margin of error—$\sigma_{\bar{x}}$ unknown

$$\pm t_{\alpha/2}\left(\text{df}\right)\frac{s_{\bar{x}}}{\sqrt{n}}\left(\text{df} = \text{degree of freedom}\right)$$

Formula 6.1d Margin of error—difference between 2 means when $\sigma_{\bar{x}}$ is known

$$\pm z_{\alpha/2}\, s_{\text{pooled}}\sqrt{\frac{1}{n_1}+\frac{1}{n_2}}$$

Formula 6.1e Margin of error—difference between 2 means when σ is unknown

$$\text{degree of freedom df} = \left(n_1 - 1\right) + \left(n_2 - 1\right)$$

$$s_{\text{pooled}=}\sqrt{\frac{\left(n_1 - 1\right)s_1^2 + \left(n_2 - 1\right)s_2^2}{n_1 + n_2 - 2}}$$

$$\pm t_{\alpha/2}\left(n_1 + n_2 - 2\right)s_{\text{pooled}}\sqrt{\frac{1}{n_1}+\frac{1}{n_2}}$$

Formula 6.1f Margin of error—proportions

$$\pm z_{\alpha/2}\sqrt{\frac{\hat{p}\left(1-\hat{p}\right)}{n}}$$

Formula 6.1g Confidence interval—continuous variables

$$\bar{x} \pm z_{\alpha/2}\text{SE} = \bar{x} \pm z_{\alpha/2}\frac{\sigma}{\sqrt{n}} \text{ if } \sigma_{\bar{x}} \text{ is unknown, replace z for t, and } \mu \text{ with } \bar{x}$$

Formula 6.1h Confidence interval—difference of 2 means

$$\bar{x}_1 - \bar{x}_2 \pm z_{\alpha/2}\, s_{\text{pooled}}\sqrt{\frac{1}{n_1}+\frac{1}{n_2}} \text{ if } n_1 \text{ or } n_2 < 30 \text{ use t instead of z}$$

Formula 6.1i Confidence interval—proportions, dichotomous variables

$$\hat{p} \pm z_{\alpha/2}\sqrt{\frac{\hat{p}\left(1-\hat{p}\right)}{n}}$$

Formula 6.1j Confidence interval—difference of 2 population proportions

$$\hat{p}_1 - \hat{p}_2 \pm z_{\alpha/2}\sqrt{\frac{\hat{p}_1\left(1-\hat{p}_1\right)}{n_1}+\frac{\hat{p}_2\left(1-\hat{p}_2\right)}{n_2}}$$

Formula 6.1k Confidence interval for an odds ratio

$$e^{\ln(\widehat{OR}) \pm z_{\alpha/2} \sqrt{\frac{1}{a} + \frac{1}{b} + \frac{1}{c} + \frac{1}{d}}}$$ (a,b,c,d—see Chapter 2 table in Appendix 1)

Formula 6.1l Confidence interval for a relative risk

$$e^{\ln(\widehat{RR}) \pm z_{\alpha/2} \sqrt{\frac{1}{a} - \frac{1}{a+b} + \frac{1}{c} - \frac{1}{c+d}}}$$ (a,b,c,d—see Chapter 3 table in Appendix 1)

Equation 6.1a

Mean $\bar{x} = 4.25$ DMFT; standard deviation $s_{\bar{x}} = 1.64$; sample $n = 83$

$$SE_{\bar{x}} = \frac{1.64}{\sqrt{83}} = 0.18$$ (Formula 4.1)

$$\pm z_{0.05/2} = \pm 1.96$$ (Formula 6.1a)

$$4.25 \pm 1.96 \times 0.18 = 4.25 \pm 0.35$$ (Formula 6.1g)

mean (95% confidence interval (CI)) 4.25 DMFT (3.90 DMFT to 4.60 DMFT)

Equation 6.1b

$$\text{Margin of error} = \pm 1.96 \times 0.18 = 0.35$$ (Formula 4.2)

Equation 6.2

The same equation as Equation 6.1a with the same confidence coefficient = 95%, the same $\bar{x} = 4.25$ DMFT, the same $s_{\bar{x}} = 1.64$, but $n = 159$, and thus $SE_{\bar{x}} = 0.13$

$$\text{mean}\left(95\% \text{ confidence interval}(CI)\right); 4.25 \text{ DMFT}\left(95\% \text{ CI}; 4.00 \text{ DMFT to } 4.50 \text{ DMFT}\right)$$

(Formula 6.1g)

Equation 6.3

The same equation as Equation 6.1a but with a confidence coefficient = 90%, the same $\bar{x} = 4.25$ DMFT, the same $s_{\bar{x}} = 1.64$, $n = 80$, $SE_{\bar{x}} = 0.18$

$$\text{A 90\% interval is the } z - \text{score between} -5.0\% \text{ and } +5.0\% = \pm z_{\alpha/2} = 1.64$$ (Formula 6.1a)

$$\text{mean}\left(90\% \text{ confidence interval}(CI)\right); 4.25 \text{ DMFT}\left(90\% \text{ CI}; 3.95 \text{ DMFT to } 4.55 \text{ DMFT}\right)$$

(Formula 6.1g)

Equation 6.4

The same equation as Equation 6.1a but with a confidence coefficient = 99%, the same $\bar{x} = 4.25$ DMFT, the same $s_{\bar{x}} = 1.64$, $n = 80$, $SE_{\bar{x}} = 0.18$

$$\text{A 99\% interval is the } z - \text{score between} -0.05\% \text{ and } +0.05\% = \pm z_{\alpha/2} = 2.58$$ (Formula 6.1a)

$$\text{mean}\left(99\% \text{ confidence interval}(CI)\right); 4.25 \text{ DMFT}\left(99\% \text{ CI}; 3.78 \text{ DMFT to } 4.72 \text{ DMFT}\right)$$

(Formula 6.1g)

Equation 6.5

The same equation as Equation 6.1a with the same confidence coefficient = 95%, the same $\bar{x} = 4.25$ DMFT, the same $s_{\bar{x}} = 1.64$, but $n = 20$, and thus $SE_{\bar{x}} = 0.37$

$$\text{mean}\left(95\% \text{ confidence interval}\left(\text{CI}\right)\right); 4.25 \, \text{DMFT}\left(95\% \, \text{CI}; 3.53 \, \text{DMFT to } 4.97 \, \text{DMFT}\right)$$

(Formula 6.1g)

Equation 6.6
The same equation as Equation 6.1a with the same confidence coefficient = 95%, the same $\bar{x} = 4.25 \, \text{DMFT}$, the same $s_{\bar{x}} = 1.64$, but n = 320, and thus $\text{SE}_{\bar{x}} = 0.09$

$$\text{mean}\left(95\% \text{ confidence interval}\left(\text{CI}\right)\right); 4.25 \, \text{DMFT}\left(95\% \, \text{CI}; 4.07 \, \text{DMFT to } 4.43 \, \text{DMFT}\right)$$

(Formula 6.1g)

Equation "Table 6.2b" Different confidence intervals (CIs) surrounding relative risk reduction (RRR) when keeping the RRR and the absolute risk difference (ARD) the same but changing sample sizes. Study 6.1 from Table 6.2.

$$\text{RR} = \frac{\dfrac{4}{4+16}}{\dfrac{6}{6+14}} = \frac{0.20}{0.30} = 0.67$$

(Formula 2.4)

$$\text{RRR} = \frac{\dfrac{4}{4+16}}{\dfrac{6}{6+14}} - 1 = \frac{0.20}{0.30} - 1 = -0.33$$

(Formula 2.6)

$$\text{ARD} = \frac{4}{4+16} - \frac{6}{6+14} = 0.20 - 0.30 = -0.10$$

(Formula 2.3)

$$95\% \, \text{CI} = 1 - e^{\ln(0.67)\pm1.96\sqrt{\left(\frac{1}{4}+\frac{1}{6}-\frac{1}{4+16}-\frac{1}{6+14}\right)}} => -1.01 \text{ to } 0.78$$

(Formula 6.1l)

Chapter 7   Understanding and interpreting power analysis and sample size

Formula 7.1 Sample size for the comparison of two means

$$n = \frac{\left(z_{\alpha/2} + z_{1-\beta}\right)^2 \times 2 \times s_{\text{pooled}}^2}{\text{size of the effect}^2}$$

Equation 7.1a Sample size for the comparison of two means

Alpha $\left(\alpha\right) = 0.05$, $s_{\text{pooled}} = 2.6$, power = 0.80, size of the effect = 10% (On a visual analog scale for pain intensity ranging from 0 to 10)

$$n = \frac{\left(1.9600 + 0.8416\right)^2 \times 2 \times 2.6^2}{1.0^2} = 107$$

(Formula 7.1)

Equation 7.1b Sample size for the comparison of two means

$$\text{Alpha} \left(\alpha \right) = 0.05, s_{\text{pooled}} = 2.6, \text{power} = 0.80, \text{size of the effect}$$
$$= \textbf{15\%} \left(\text{same as } 7.1a, \text{except for the change in effect size} \right)$$

$$n = \frac{\left(1.9600 + 0.8416 \right)^2 \times 2 \times 2.6^2}{1.5^2} = 48 \tag{Formula 7.1}$$

Equation 7.2 Sample size for the comparison of two means

$$\text{Alpha} \left(\alpha \right) = \textbf{0.01}, s_{\text{pooled}} = 2.6, \text{power} = 0.80, \text{size of the effect}$$
$$= 10\% \left(\text{same as } 7.1a, \text{except for the change in alpha} \right)$$

$$n = \frac{\left(2.3263 + 0.8416 \right)^2 \times 2 \times 2.6^2}{1.0^2} = 136 \tag{Formula 7.1}$$

Equation 7.3 Sample size for the comparison of two means

$$\text{Alpha} \left(\alpha \right) = 0.05, s_{\text{pooled}} = 2.6, \text{power} = \textbf{0.90}, \text{size of the effect}$$
$$= 10\% \left(\text{same as } 7.1a, \text{except for the change in power} \right)$$

$$n = \frac{\left(1.9600 + \textbf{1.2816} \right)^2 \times 2 \times 2.6^2}{1.0^2} = 143 \tag{Formula 7.1}$$

Chapter 8　Understanding and interpreting survival analysis

Formula 8.1 General terms for a cumulative probability in survival analysis

S_t = Proportion of individuals who survived to the previous (first) interval
P_{t+1} = Proportion of individuals who survive to the current (second) interval
S_{t+1} = Proportion of individuals who survived to the current interval, given that they also survived to the previous interval (cumulative survival probability)

$$S_{t+1} = p_{t+1} \times S_t$$

Formula 8.2 Survival rate for a survival curve across three interval times

$$\textit{Survival rate} = \left(1 - \textit{hazard rate} \right) = \left(1 - \frac{\textit{dead}}{\textit{alive}} \right)$$

Survival rate at a specific time point

$$\textit{Survival rate} \left(t_3 \right) = \left(1 - \frac{\textit{dead}_{t=0}}{\textit{alive}_{t=0}} \right) x \left(1 - \frac{\textit{dead}_{t=1}}{\textit{alive}_{t=1}} \right) x \left(1 - \frac{\textit{dead}_{t=2}}{\textit{alive}_{t=2}} \right) x \left(1 - \frac{\textit{dead}_{t=3}}{\textit{alive}_{t=3}} \right)$$

Equation 8.1 Cumulative probability for interval 1

$$S_{t+1} = \left(\frac{100}{100} \right) \times \left(\frac{90}{100} \right) = 0.90 \text{ or } 90\% \tag{Formula 8.1}$$

Chapter 9   Understanding and interpreting a probabilistic-based diagnosis

	Disease present	Disease absence	
Test positive	TP	FP	TP+FP
Test negative	FN	TN	FN+TN
	TP+FN	FP+TN	TP+FP+FN+TN

TP—true positive; FN—false negative; FP—false positive, TN—true negative

Formula 9.1 Sensitivity, or true positive rate (TPR)

$$\text{sensitivity}\left(\text{TPR}\right)=\frac{\sum\text{True Positive}}{\sum\text{Disease present}}=\frac{TP}{TP+FN}$$

Formula 9.2 False negative rate (FNR)

$$\text{FNR}=\frac{\sum\text{False negative}}{\sum\text{Disease present}}=\frac{FN}{TP+FN}=1-\text{sensitivity}$$

Formula 9.3 Specificity, or true negative rate (TNR)

$$\text{specificity}\left(\text{TNR}\right)=\frac{\sum\text{True negative}}{\sum\text{Disease absent}}=\frac{TN}{TN+FP}$$

Formula 9.4 False positive rate (FPR)

$$\text{FPR}=\frac{\sum\text{False positive}}{\sum\text{Disease absent}}=\frac{FP}{TN+FP}=1-\text{specificity}$$

Formula 9.5 Positive predictive value (PPV), knowing test result values

$$\text{PPV}=\frac{\sum\text{True postive}}{\sum\text{Test outcome positive}}=\frac{TP}{TP+FP}$$

Formula 9.6 Negative predictive value (NPV), knowing test results

$$\text{NPV}=\frac{\sum\text{True negative}}{\sum\text{Test outcome negative}}=\frac{TN}{TN+FN}$$

Formula 9.7 Test accuracy

$$\text{accuracy}=\frac{\sum\text{True positive}+\sum\text{True negative}}{\sum\text{total population}}=\frac{TP+TN}{TP+FN+TN+FP}$$

Formula 9.8 Positive predictive value (PPV), knowing only prevalence, sensitivity, and specificity

$$\text{PPV}=\frac{\text{sensitivity}\times\text{prevalence}}{\left(\text{sensitivity}\times\text{prevalence}\right)+\left(\left(1-\text{specificity}\right)\times\left(1-\text{prevalence}\right)\right)}$$

Formula 9.9 Positive likelihood ratio (LR^+)

$$LR^+ = \frac{\text{True positive rate}}{\text{False positive rate}} = \frac{\text{sensitivity}}{1-\text{specificity}} = \frac{\dfrac{TP}{TP+FN}}{\dfrac{FP}{FP+TN}}$$

Formula 9.10 Negative likelihood ratio (LR^-)

$$LR^- = \frac{\text{False negative rate}}{\text{True negative rate}} = \frac{1-\text{sensitivity}}{\text{specificity}} = \frac{\dfrac{FN}{TP+FN}}{\dfrac{TN}{FP+TN}}$$

Formula 9.11 Transforming probabilities to odds

$$\frac{\text{probability}}{1-\text{probability}} = \frac{P(X)}{1-P(X)} = \text{odds}$$

Formula 9.12 Transforming pretest odds to posttest odds

$$\text{Posttest odds} = LR^+ \times \text{pretest odds}$$

Formula 9.13 Transforming odds to probabilities

$$\frac{\text{odds}}{1+\text{odds}} = P(X) = \text{probability}$$

Formula 9.14 Direct calculation of a posttest (posterior) probability

$$LR \times \text{pretest}(\text{prior})\text{ probability} = \text{posttest}(\text{posterior})\text{ probability}$$

Formula 9.15 Posttest probability knowing the pretest probability, the sensitivity and specificity

$$\text{posttest probability} = \frac{\dfrac{\text{pretest probability}}{1-\text{pretest probability}} \times \dfrac{\text{sensitivity}}{1-\text{specificity}}}{1+\dfrac{\text{pretest probability}}{1-\text{pretest probability}} \times \dfrac{\text{sensitivity}}{1-\text{specificity}}}$$

Formula 9.16a Posttest probability knowing the pretest probability and LR^+

$$\text{posttest probability} = \frac{\dfrac{\text{pretest probability}}{1-\text{pretest probability}} \times LR^+}{1+\dfrac{\text{pretest probability}}{1-\text{pretest probability}} \times LR^+}$$

Formula 9.16b Posttest probability knowing the pretest probability and LR^-

$$\text{posttest probability} = \frac{\dfrac{\text{pretest probability}}{1-\text{pretest probability}} \times LR^-}{1+\dfrac{\text{pretest probability}}{1-\text{pretest probability}} \times LR^-}$$

Equations Table 9.2

	Disease present	Disease absent	Total
Test positive	285 (TP)	970 (FP)	1,255
Test negative	15 (FN)	8,730 (TN)	8,745
Total	300	9,700	10,000

TP—true positive; FN—false negative; FP—false positive, TN—true negative
TPR- true positive rate; FNR- false negative rate; TNR—true negative rate; FPR—false positive rate

Equation 9.1. Sensitivity, or true positive rate (TPR)

$$\text{sensitivity (TPR)} = \frac{285}{300} = 0.95 = 95\% \qquad \text{(Formula 9.1)}$$

Equation 9.2. False negative rate (FNR)

$$\text{FNR} \frac{\text{FN}}{\text{TP} + \text{FN}} = \frac{15}{300} = 0.05 = 5\% \qquad \text{(Formula 9.2)}$$

$$\text{FNR} = 1 - 95\% = 5\% \qquad \text{(Formula 9.2)}$$

Equation 9.3. Specificity, or true negative rate

$$\text{specificity (TNR)} = \frac{8,730}{9,700} = 0.90 = 90\% \qquad \text{(Formula 9.3)}$$

Equation 9.4. False positive rate (FPR)

$$\text{FPR} = \frac{970}{9,700} = 0.10 = 10\% $$

$$\text{FPR} = 1 - 90\% = 10\% \qquad \text{(Formula 9.4)}$$

Equation 9.5. Positive predictive value (PPV), knowing test result values

$$\text{PPV} = \frac{285}{1,255} = 0.227 = 22.7\% \qquad \text{(Formula 9.5)}$$

Equation 9.6. Negative predictive value (NPV), knowing the test result values

$$\text{NPV} = \frac{8,730}{8,745} = 0.998 = 99.8\% \qquad \text{(Formula 9.6)}$$

Equation 9.7a. Test accuracy

$$\text{accuracy} = \frac{9,015}{10,000} = 0.9015 = 90.15\% \qquad \text{(Formula 9.7)}$$

Equation 9.7b. Test accuracy—flawed reflection of a test's accuracy (very low sensitivity yet high accuracy)

> Hypothetical example—total population $= 10,000$, prevalence $= 3\%$, test sensitivity $= 5\%$, test specificity $= 99\%$. Based on these values —TP $= 15$, TN $= 9,603$, FN $= 285$, FP $= 97$

$$\text{accuracy} = \frac{9,618}{10,000} = 0.9618 = 96.18\% \tag{Formula 9.7}$$

Equation 9.8a Positive predictive value (PPV), knowing only prevalence, sensitivity, and specificity

$$\text{PPV} = \frac{0.95 \times 0.03}{\left(0.95 \times 0.03\right) + \left(\left(1 - 0.90\right) \times \left(1 - 0.03\right)\right)} = 0.227 = 22.7\% \tag{Formula 9.8}$$

Equation 9.8b Positive predictive value (PPV), knowing only prevalence, sensitivity, and specificity

$$\text{PPV} = \frac{0.95 \times 0.05}{\left(0.95 \times 0.05\right) + \left(\left(1 - 0.90\right) \times \left(1 - 0.05\right)\right)} = 0.333 = 33.3\% \tag{Formula 9.8}$$

Equation 9.9. Positive likelihood ratio (LR^+)

$$\text{LR}^+ = \frac{0.95}{1 - 0.90} = \frac{0.95}{0.10} = 9.50 \text{ , or}$$

$$\text{LR}^+ = \frac{\dfrac{285}{285 + 15}}{\dfrac{970}{970 + 8,730}} = \frac{0.95}{0.10} = 9.50 \tag{Formula 9.9}$$

Equation 9.10. Negative likelihood ratio (LR^-)

$$\text{LR}^- = \frac{1 - 0.95}{0.90} = \frac{0.05}{0.90} = 0.06 \text{ , or}$$

$$\text{LR}^- = \frac{\dfrac{15}{285 + 15}}{\dfrac{8,730}{970 + 8,730}} = \frac{0.05}{0.90} = 0.06 \tag{Formula 9.10}$$

Equation 9.11a. Calculating posttest probabilities with different pretest probabilities

Pretest probability $= 40\%$, test sensitivity $= 80\%$, test specificity $= 80\%$

$$\text{Transforming pretest probability to pretest odds} - \frac{0.40}{1 - 0.40} = \frac{0.40}{0.60} = 0.667 \tag{Formula 9.11}$$

$$\text{Positive likelihood ratio } (\text{LR}^+) - \text{LR}^+ = \frac{0.80}{1 - 0.80} = \frac{0.80}{0.20} = 4.00 \tag{Formula 9.9}$$

$$\text{Posttest odds} = 4.00 \times 0.667 = 2.668 \tag{Formula 9.12}$$

$$\text{Transforming posttest odds to posttest probability} - \frac{2.668}{1 + 2.668} = \frac{2.668}{3.668} = 0.727 = 72.7\% \tag{Formula 9.13}$$

Equation 9.11b.
Pretest probability = 10%, test sensitivity = 80%, test specificity = 80%

$$\text{Transforming pretest probability to pretest odds} - \frac{0.10}{1-0.10} = \frac{0.10}{0.90} = 0.111 \qquad \text{(Formula 9.11)}$$

$$\text{Positive likelihood ratio} \left(\text{LR}+\right) - \text{LR}^+ = \frac{0.80}{1-0.80} = \frac{0.80}{0.20} = 4.00 \qquad \text{(Formula 9.9)}$$

$$\text{Posttest odds} = 4.00 \times 0.111 = 0.444 \qquad \text{(Formula 9.12)}$$

$$\text{Transforming posttest odds to posttest probability} - \frac{0.444}{1+0.444} = \frac{0.444}{1.444} = 0.307 = 30.7\%$$

$$\text{(Formula 9.13)}$$

Chapter 11   Understanding and interpreting regression analysis

Formula 11.1 Linear formula

$$y = bx + a$$

Formula 11.2 Simple linear regression model

$$y = \beta_0 + \beta_1 x_1 + \varepsilon$$

Formula 11.3 Logistic model to estimate probability (risk)

$$P(X) = \frac{1}{1 + e^{-(\beta_0 + \beta_1 X_1 + \beta_2 X_2 + \dots \beta_i X_i)}} = \frac{e^{(\beta_0 + \beta_1 X_1 + \beta_2 X_2 + \dots \beta_i X_i)}}{1 + e^{(\beta_0 + \beta_1 X_1 + \beta_2 X_2 + \dots \beta_i X_i)}}$$

Formula 11.4 Logit transformation of logistic model

$$\text{Logit } P(X) = \ln\left[\text{Odds}\right] = \ln\left[\frac{P(X)}{1-P(X)}\right] = \ln\left[\frac{\frac{1}{1 + e^{-(\beta_0 + \beta_1 X_1 + \beta_2 X_2 + \dots \beta_i X_i)}}}{1 - \frac{1}{1 + e^{-(\beta_0 + \beta_1 X_1 + \beta_2 X_2 + \dots \beta_i X_i)}}}\right] = \beta_0 + \beta_1 X_1 + \beta_2 X_2 + \dots \beta_i X_i$$

The logit is equal to the natural logarithm of the odds and is also known as "log-odds."
Formula 11.5 Converting the log-odds (i.e., the ln(odds) to odds)

$$\text{Odds} = e^{\ln\left[\text{Odds}\right]} = e^{\left[\beta_0 + \beta_1 X_1 + \beta_2 X_2 + \dots \beta_i X_i\right]}$$

Formula 11.6 Estimating the crude OR and 95% confidence interval (CI) with logistic regression coefficients and standard error (SE) for the coefficient

$$\widehat{\text{OR}} = e^{\hat{\beta}_i}$$

$$95\% \text{ CI} = \widehat{\text{OR}} \pm 1.96 \times \text{SE}$$

Equation 11.1 The expected value of a population mean after estimating regression coefficients with simple linear regression

$$\hat{y}_i = -54.2 + (0.73 \times 185\,\text{cm.}) = 80.85\,\text{kg} \qquad \text{(Formula 11.2)}$$

Equation 11.2 "Table 11.1" Estimating odds for a person

$$ln\left[\widehat{Odds}\right] = -3.12 \times (constant) + 3.21 \times (smoking) + 1.68 \times (alcohol) + 1.62 \times (CVD)$$
$$+ 2.92 \times (diabetes) - 2.33 \times (brushing)$$

Person #1: smoking = yes, alcohol use = yes, cardiovascular disease = yes, toothbrushing = yes

$$ln\left[\widehat{Odds}\right] = -3.12 + 3.21 \times (1) + 1.68 \times (1) + 1.62 \times (1) + 2.92 \times (1)$$
$$- 2.33 \times (1) = 3.98 \tag{Formula 11.4}$$

$$\widehat{Odds} = e^{3.98} = 53.52 \tag{Formula 11.5}$$

Person #2: smoking = no, alcohol use = no, cardiovascular disease = yes, toothbrushing = yes.

$$ln\left[\widehat{Odds}\right] = -3.12 + 3.21 \times (0) + 1.68 \times (0) + 1.62 \times (1) + 2.92 \times (0) - 2.33 \times (1) = -3.83$$

$$\tag{Formula 11.4}$$

$$\widehat{Odds} = e^{-3.83} = 0.022 \tag{Formula 11.5}$$

Equation 11.3 Converting odds to probability (risk)

$$Person\#1 : P\left(\widehat{X}\right) = \widehat{Risk} = \frac{53.52}{1 + 53.52} = \frac{53.52}{54.52} = 0.9817 \text{ or } 98.17\% \tag{Formula 9.13}$$

$$Person\#2 : P\left(\widehat{X}\right) = \widehat{Risk} = \frac{0.022}{1 + 0.022} = \frac{0.022}{1.022} = 0.0215 \text{ or } 2.15\% \tag{Formula 9.13}$$

Equation 11.5—Estimating the crude OR with a logistic regression coefficient

$$\widehat{OR} = e^{-0.5} = 0.61 \tag{Formula 11.6}$$

Chapter 14 Understanding and interpreting patient-reported outcomes

Formula 14.1 Cohen's kappa (chance-corrected agreement)

$$k = \frac{\text{Observed agreement} - \text{Expected agreement*}}{1 - \text{Expected agreement}}$$

*50% is always used for the expected agreement.

Equation 14.1 Comparison of raw agreement (80%) and the Cohen's kappa statistic or chance-corrected agreement (60%).

$$k = \frac{\frac{80}{100} - \frac{50}{100}}{1 - \frac{50}{100}} = 0.60 \text{ or } 60\% \tag{Formula 14.1}$$

Chapter 15   Understanding and interpreting a cross-sectional study

	Condition present		Condition absent		Total	
Exposure present (exposed)	Exposed individuals with the condition.	a	Exposed individuals without the condition.	b	Total number of individuals exposed	a+b
Exposure absent (unexposed)	Unexposed individuals with the condition.	c	Unexposed individuals without the condition.	d	Total number of individuals unexposed	c+d
Total	Total number of individuals with the condition	a+c	Total number of individuals without the condition	b+d	Total number of individuals	a+b+c+d

Formula 15.1 Prevalence of condition among the population of interest

$$\text{Prevalence}_{\text{population}} = \frac{\text{total number of individuals with the condition}}{\text{total number of individuals}} = \frac{a+c}{a+b+c+d}$$

Formula 15.2 Prevalence of condition among exposed individuals

$$\text{Prevalence}_{\text{exposed}} = \frac{\text{exposed individuals with the condition}}{\text{total number of individuals exposed}} = \frac{a}{a+b}$$

Formula 15.3 Prevalence of condition among unexposed individuals

$$\text{Prevalence}_{\text{unexposed}} = \frac{\text{unexposed individuals with the condition}}{\text{total number of individuals unexposed}} = \frac{c}{c+d}$$

Equation 15.1 Overall prevalence in the population

$$\text{Prevalence}_{\text{population}} = \frac{100+100}{100+400+100+1,400} = 0.10 \text{ or } 10\% \qquad \text{(Formula 15.1)}$$

Equation 15.2 Prevalence of condition among exposed individuals

$$\text{Prevalence}_{\text{unexposed}} = \frac{100}{100+400} = 0.20 \text{ or } 20\% \qquad \text{(Formula 15.2)}$$

Equation 15.3 Prevalence of condition among unexposed individuals

$$\text{Prevalence}_{\text{exposed}} = \frac{100}{100+1,400} = 0.067 \text{ or } 6.7\% \qquad \text{(Formula 15.3)}$$

Equation 15.4 Prevalence odds ratio (POR)

$$\text{POR} = \frac{100\times1,400}{400\times100} = 3.5 \qquad \text{(Formula 2.8a, 2.8b, and 2.9)}$$

Equation 15.5 Prevalence ratio (exposed/unexposed)

$$\text{Prevalence ratio} = \frac{\dfrac{100}{100+400}}{\dfrac{100}{100+1,400}} = 3.0 \qquad \text{(Formula 2.4)}$$

Chapter 17   Understanding and interpreting a cohort study

Formula 17.1 Cumulative incidence/incidence proportion

$$\text{Cumulative incidence} = \frac{\text{number of individuals who develop the outomce}}{\text{total number of individuals at risk}}$$

Formula 17.2 Rate/incidence rate

$$\text{Rate} = \frac{\text{number of individuals who develop the outcome}}{\text{person-time at risk}}$$

Equation 17.1. Cumulative incidence/incidence proportion

$$\text{Cumulative incidence} = \frac{10}{100} = 0.10 \text{ or } 10\% \qquad \text{(Formula 17.1)}$$

Equation 17.2

$$\text{Rate} = \frac{10}{100\,\text{person} - \text{years} + 95\,\text{person} - \text{years}} = \frac{10}{195\,\text{person} - \text{years}} \qquad \text{(Formula 17.2)}$$
$$= 0.052 \text{ or } 5.2 \text{ per } 100\,\text{person} - \text{years}$$

Chapter 18   Understanding and interpreting a randomized controlled trial

Equation 18.1a Relative risk (RR) (treatment relative to control) for composite outcome (stroke or death)

$$\text{RR} = \frac{\dfrac{16}{16+84}}{\dfrac{26}{26+74}} = 0.62 \qquad \text{(Formula 2.4)}$$

Equation 18.1b Relative risk (RR) (treatment relative to control) for death outcome

$$\text{RR} = \frac{\dfrac{1}{1+99}}{\dfrac{1}{1+99}} = 1.00 \qquad \text{(Formula 2.4)}$$

Equation 18.1c Relative risk (RR) (treatment relative to control) for stroke outcome

$$RR = \dfrac{\dfrac{15}{15+85}}{\dfrac{25}{25+75}} = 0.60 \qquad\qquad \text{(Formula 2.4)}$$

Equation 18.2a Relative risk (RR) (treatment relative to control),
Study A, ignore lost to follow-up:

$$RR = \dfrac{\dfrac{20}{20+80}}{\dfrac{40}{40+100}} = 0.50 \qquad\qquad \text{(Formula 2.4)}$$

Study A, worse-case scenario:

$$RR\,\dfrac{\dfrac{22}{22+77}}{\dfrac{40}{40+100}} = 0.55 \qquad\qquad \text{(Formula 2.4)}$$

Equation 18.2b Relative risk (RR) (treatment relative to control),
Study B, ignore lost to follow-up:

$$RR = \dfrac{\dfrac{2}{2+99}}{\dfrac{4}{4+96}} = 0.50 \qquad\qquad \text{(Formula 2.4)}$$

Study B, worse-case scenario:

$$RR = \dfrac{\dfrac{4}{4+96}}{\dfrac{4}{4+96}} = 1.00 \qquad\qquad \text{(Formula 2.4)}$$

Equation 18.3a Relative risk (RR) (treatment relative to control), no subgroup

$$RR = \dfrac{\dfrac{50}{50+450}}{\dfrac{200}{200+300}} = 0.25 \qquad\qquad \text{(Formula 2.4)}$$

Equation 18.3b 95% Confidence interval for a relative risk (RR) (treatment relative to control), no subgroup.

$$\text{95\% CI for a relative risk} = e^{\ln(0.25)\pm1.96\sqrt{\frac{1}{50}-\frac{1}{50+450}+\frac{1}{200}-\frac{1}{200+300}}} = 0.19, 0.33 \qquad \text{(Formula 6.11)}$$

Equation 18.3c Relative risk (RR) (treatment relative to control), subgroup: mutation A

$$RR = \dfrac{AR_{exposure}}{AR_{control}} = \dfrac{\dfrac{a}{a+b}}{\dfrac{c}{c+d}} = \dfrac{\dfrac{5}{5+120}}{\dfrac{50}{50+75}} = 0.10$$

Equation 18.3d 95% CI for a relative risk; subgroup: mutation A

$$95\% \text{ CI for a relative risk} = e^{\ln(0.10)\pm1.96\sqrt{\frac{1}{5}-\frac{1}{5+120}+\frac{1}{50}-\frac{1}{50+75}}} = 0.04, 0.24 \qquad \text{(Formula 6.1l)}$$

Equation 18.3e Relative risk (RR) (treatment relative to control), subgroup: mutation B

$$\text{RR} = \frac{\dfrac{20}{20+105}}{\dfrac{50}{50+75}} = 0.40 \qquad \text{(Formula 2.4)}$$

Equation 18.3f 95% CI for a relative risk; subgroup: mutation B

$$95\% \text{ CI for a relative risk} = e^{\ln(0.40)\pm1.96\sqrt{\frac{1}{20}-\frac{1}{20+105}+\frac{1}{50}-\frac{1}{50+75}}} = 0.25, 0.63 \qquad \text{(Formula 6.1l)}$$

Chapter 19   Understanding and interpreting meta-analysis

Formula 19.1 Pooled effect estimate

$$\theta = \frac{\Sigma W_i Y_i}{\Sigma W_i}$$

Formula 19.2 Inverse-variance method to weigh studies in a fixed effect meta-analysis

$$W_i = \frac{1}{SE_i^2}$$

Formula 19.3 Inverse-variance method to weigh studies in a random effects meta-analysis

$$W_i = \frac{1}{SE_i^2 + \tau^2}$$

Appendix 2

Z-table

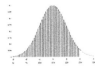
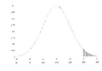
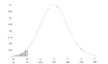
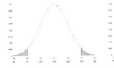

| z-score of +1.96 (0.9750 (97.5%)), which covers an area under the curve of **97.5%** | 1 less the z-score of +1.96 (1 (100%) − 0.9750 (97.5%) = 0.0250 (2.5%)), which covers an area under the curve of **2.5%** | z-score of −1.96 *symmetrical to 1 less the z-score of +1.96* (1 (100%) − 0.9750 (97.5%)) = 0.0250 (2.5%)), which covers an area under the curve of **2.5%** | z-score of −1.96 less the z-score of +1.96 2.5% + 2.5% = **5.0%** | z-score between +1.96 and −1.96 (0.9750 (97.5%) − (1 (100%) − 0.9750 (97.5%))) or 2 × (0.9750 (97.5%) − 1) = 0.9500 (95%)), which covers an area under the curve of **95%** |

Probability content from −∞ to z

z	.00	.01	.02	.03	.04	.05	.06	.07	.08	.09
.0	0.5000	0.5040	0.5080	0.5120	0.5160	0.5199	0.5239	0.5279	0.5319	0.5359
.1	0.5398	0.5438	0.5478	0.5517	0.5557	0.5596	0.5636	0.5675	0.5714	0.5753
.2	0.5793	0.5832	0.5871	0.5910	0.5948	0.5987	0.6026	0.6064	0.6103	0.6141
.3	0.6179	0.6217	0.6255	0.6293	0.6331	0.6368	0.6406	0.6443	0.6480	0.6517
.4	0.6554	0.6591	0.6628	0.6664	0.6700	0.6736	0.6772	0.6808	0.6844	0.6879
.5	0.6915	0.6950	0.6985	0.7019	0.7054	0.7088	0.7123	0.7157	0.7190	0.7224
.6	0.7257	0.7291	0.7324	0.7357	0.7389	0.7422	0.7454	0.7486	0.7517	0.7549
.7	0.7580	0.7611	0.7642	0.7673	0.7704	0.7734	0.7764	0.7794	0.7823	0.7852
.8	0.7881	0.7910	0.7939	0.7967	0.7995	0.8023	0.8051	0.8078	0.8106	0.8133
.9	0.8159	0.8186	0.8212	0.8238	0.8264	0.8289	0.8315	0.8340	0.8365	0.8389
1.0	0.8413	0.8438	0.8461	0.8485	0.8508	0.8531	0.8554	0.8577	0.8599	0.8621
1.1	0.8643	0.8665	0.8686	0.8708	0.8729	0.8749	0.8770	0.8790	0.8810	0.8830

(Continued)

Statistics for Dental Clinicians, First Edition. Michael Glick, Alonso Carrasco-Labra, and Olivia Urquhart.
© 2024 John Wiley & Sons, Inc. Published 2024 by John Wiley & Sons, Inc.

z	.00	.01	.02	.03	.04	.05	.06	.07	.08	.09
1.2	0.8849	0.8869	0.8888	0.8907	0.8925	0.8944	0.8962	0.8980	0.8997	0.9015
1.3	0.9032	0.9049	0.9066	0.9082	0.9099	0.9115	0.9131	0.9147	0.9162	0.9177
1.4	0.9192	0.9207	0.9222	0.9236	0.9251	0.9265	0.9279	0.9292	0.9306	0.9319
1.5	0.9332	0.9345	0.9357	0.9370	0.9382	0.9394	0.9406	0.9418	0.9429	0.9441
1.6	0.9452	0.9463	0.9474	0.9484	0.9495	0.9505	0.9515	0.9525	0.9535	0.9545
1.7	0.9554	0.9564	0.9573	0.9582	0.9591	0.9599	0.9608	0.9616	0.9625	0.9633
1.8	0.9641	0.9649	0.9656	0.9664	0.9671	0.9678	0.9686	0.9693	0.9699	0.9706
1.9	0.9713	0.9719	0.9726	0.9732	0.9738	0.9744	0.9750	0.9756	0.9761	0.9767
2.0	0.9772	0.9778	0.9783	0.9788	0.9793	0.9798	0.9803	0.9808	0.9812	0.9817
2.1	0.9821	0.9826	0.9830	0.9834	0.9838	0.9842	0.9846	0.9850	0.9854	0.9857
2.2	0.9861	0.9864	0.9868	0.9871	0.9875	0.9878	0.9881	0.9884	0.9887	0.9890
2.3	0.9893	0.9896	0.9898	0.9901	0.9904	0.9906	0.9909	0.9911	0.9913	0.9916
2.4	0.9918	0.9920	0.9922	0.9925	0.9927	0.9929	0.9931	0.9932	0.9934	0.9936
2.5	0.9938	0.9940	0.9941	0.9943	0.9945	0.9946	0.9948	0.9949	0.9951	0.9952
2.6	0.9953	0.9955	0.9956	0.9957	0.9959	0.9960	0.9961	0.9962	0.9963	0.9964
2.7	0.9965	0.9966	0.9967	0.9968	0.9969	0.9970	0.9971	0.9972	0.9973	0.9974
2.8	0.9974	0.9975	0.9976	0.9977	0.9977	0.9978	0.9979	0.9979	0.9980	0.9981
2.9	0.9981	0.9982	0.9982	0.9983	0.9984	0.9984	0.9985	0.9985	0.9986	0.9986
3.0	0.9987	0.9987	0.9987	0.9988	0.9988	0.9989	0.9989	0.9989	0.9990	0.9990

Example. A z-score of 2.06 equals 0.9803 (98.03%) (see highlighted cell) (Appendix 1, Equation 5.2)

Appendix 3

T-table

1-tail	0.25	0.20	0.15	0.1	0.05	0.025	0.01	0.005	0.001	0.0005
2-tail	0.50	0.40	0.30	0.2	0.1	0.05	0.02	0.01	0.002	0.001
df										
1	1.000	1.376	1.963	3.078	6.314	12.706	31.821	63.657	318.309	636.619
2	0.816	1.061	1.386	1.886	2.920	4.303	6.965	9.925	22.327	31.599
3	0.765	0.978	1.250	1.638	2.353	3.182	4.541	5.841	10.215	12.924
4	0.741	0.941	1.190	1.533	2.132	2.776	3.747	4.604	7.173	8.610
5	0.727	0.920	1.156	1.476	2.015	2.571	3.365	4.032	5.893	6.869
6	0.718	0.906	1.134	1.440	1.943	2.447	3.143	3.707	5.208	5.959
7	0.711	0.896	1.119	1.415	1.895	2.365	2.998	3.499	4.785	5.408
8	0.706	0.889	1.108	1.397	1.860	2.306	2.896	3.355	4.501	5.041
9	0.703	0.883	1.100	1.383	1.833	2.262	2.821	3.250	4.297	4.781
10	0.700	0.879	1.093	1.372	1.812	2.228	2.764	3.169	4.144	4.587
11	0.697	0.876	1.088	1.363	1.796	2.201	2.718	3.106	4.025	4.437
12	0.695	0.873	1.083	1.356	1.782	2.179	2.681	3.055	3.930	4.318
13	0.694	0.870	1.079	1.350	1.771	2.160	2.650	3.012	3.852	4.221
14	0.692	0.868	1.076	1.345	1.761	2.145	2.624	2.977	3.787	4.140
15	0.691	0.866	1.074	1.341	1.753	2.131	2.602	2.947	3.733	4.073
16	0.690	0.865	1.071	1.337	1.746	2.120	2.583	2.921	3.686	4.015
17	0.689	0.863	1.069	1.333	1.740	2.110	2.567	2.898	3.646	3.965
18	0.688	0.862	1.067	1.330	1.734	2.101	2.552	2.878	3.610	3.922
19	0.688	0.861	1.066	1.328	1.729	2.093	2.539	2.861	3.579	3.883
20	0.687	0.860	1.064	1.325	1.725	2.086	2.528	2.845	3.552	3.850
21	0.686	0.859	1.063	1.323	1.721	2.080	2.518	2.831	3.527	3.819
22	0.686	0.858	1.061	1.321	1.717	2.074	2.508	2.819	3.505	3.792
23	0.685	0.858	1.060	1.319	1.714	2.069	2.500	2.807	3.485	3.768
24	0.685	0.857	1.059	1.318	1.711	2.064	2.492	2.797	3.467	3.745
25	0.684	0.856	1.058	1.316	1.708	2.060	2.485	2.787	3.450	3.725

(Continued)

Statistics for Dental Clinicians, First Edition. Michael Glick, Alonso Carrasco-Labra, and Olivia Urquhart.
© 2024 John Wiley & Sons, Inc. Published 2024 by John Wiley & Sons, Inc.

(Continued)

26	0.684	0.856	1.058	1.315	1.706	2.056	2.479	2.779	3.435	3.707
27	0.684	0.855	1.057	1.314	1.703	2.052	2.473	2.771	3.421	3.690
28	0.683	0.855	1.056	1.313	1.701	2.048	2.467	2.763	3.408	3.674
29	0.683	0.854	1.055	1.311	1.699	2.045	2.462	2.756	3.396	3.659
30	0.683	0.854	1.055	1.310	1.697	2.042	2.457	2.750	3.385	3.646
31	0.682	0.853	1.054	1.309	1.696	2.040	2.453	2.744	3.375	3.633
32	0.682	0.853	1.054	1.309	1.694	2.037	2.449	2.738	3.365	3.622
33	0.682	0.853	1.053	1.308	1.692	2.035	2.445	2.733	3.356	3.611
34	0.682	0.852	1.052	1.307	1.691	2.032	2.441	2.728	3.348	3.601
35	0.682	0.852	1.052	1.306	1.690	2.030	2.438	2.724	3.340	3.591
36	0.681	0.852	1.052	1.306	1.688	2.028	2.434	2.719	3.333	3.582
37	0.681	0.851	1.051	1.305	1.687	2.026	2.431	2.715	3.326	3.574
38	0.681	0.851	1.051	1.304	1.686	2.024	2.429	2.712	3.319	3.566
39	0.681	0.851	1.050	1.304	1.685	2.023	2.426	2.708	3.313	3.558
40	0.681	0.851	1.050	1.303	1.684	2.021	2.423	2.704	3.307	3.551
41	0.681	0.850	1.050	1.303	1.683	2.020	2.421	2.701	3.301	3.544
42	0.680	0.850	1.049	1.302	1.682	2.018	2.418	2.698	3.296	3.538
43	0.680	0.850	1.049	1.302	1.681	2.017	2.416	2.695	3.291	3.532
44	0.680	0.850	1.049	1.301	1.680	2.015	2.414	2.692	3.286	3.526
45	0.680	0.850	1.049	1.301	1.679	2.014	2.412	2.690	3.281	3.520
46	0.680	0.850	1.048	1.300	1.679	2.013	2.410	2.687	3.277	3.515
47	0.680	0.849	1.048	1.300	1.678	2.012	2.408	2.685	3.273	3.510
48	0.680	0.849	1.048	1.299	1.677	2.011	2.407	2.682	3.269	3.505
49	0.680	0.849	1.048	1.299	1.677	2.010	2.405	2.680	3.265	3.500
50	0.679	0.849	1.047	1.299	1.676	2.009	2.403	2.678	3.261	3.496
51	0.679	0.849	1.047	1.298	1.675	2.008	2.402	2.676	3.258	3.492
52	0.679	0.849	1.047	1.298	1.675	2.007	2.400	2.674	3.255	3.488
53	0.679	0.848	1.047	1.298	1.674	2.006	2.399	2.672	3.251	3.484
54	0.679	0.848	1.046	1.297	1.674	2.005	2.397	2.670	3.248	3.480
55	0.679	0.848	1.046	1.297	1.673	2.004	2.396	2.668	3.245	3.476
56	0.679	0.848	1.046	1.297	1.673	2.003	2.395	2.667	3.242	3.473
57	0.679	0.848	1.046	1.297	1.672	2.002	2.394	2.665	3.239	3.470
58	0.679	0.848	1.046	1.296	1.672	2.002	2.392	2.663	3.237	3.466
59	0.679	0.848	1.046	1.296	1.671	2.001	2.391	2.662	3.234	3.463
60	0.679	0.848	1.045	1.296	1.671	2.000	2.390	2.660	3.232	3.460
61	0.679	0.848	1.045	1.296	1.670	2.000	2.389	2.659	3.229	3.457
62	0.678	0.847	1.045	1.295	1.670	1.999	2.388	2.657	3.227	3.454
63	0.678	0.847	1.045	1.295	1.669	1.998	2.387	2.656	3.225	3.452
64	0.678	0.847	1.045	1.295	1.669	1.998	2.386	2.655	3.223	3.449
65	0.678	0.847	1.045	1.295	1.669	1.997	2.385	2.654	3.220	3.447

66	0.678	0.847	1.045	1.295	1.668	1.997	2.384	2.652	3.218	3.444
67	0.678	0.847	1.045	1.294	1.668	1.996	2.383	2.651	3.216	3.442
68	0.678	0.847	1.044	1.294	1.668	1.995	2.382	2.650	3.214	3.439
69	0.678	0.847	1.044	1.294	1.667	1.995	2.382	2.649	3.213	3.437
70	0.678	0.847	1.044	1.294	1.667	1.994	2.381	2.648	3.211	3.435
71	0.678	0.847	1.044	1.294	1.667	1.994	2.380	2.647	3.209	3.433
72	0.678	0.847	1.044	1.293	1.666	1.993	2.379	2.646	3.207	3.431
73	0.678	0.847	1.044	1.293	1.666	1.993	2.379	2.645	3.206	3.429
74	0.678	0.847	1.044	1.293	1.666	1.993	2.378	2.644	3.204	3.427
75	0.678	0.846	1.044	1.293	1.665	1.992	2.377	2.643	3.202	3.425
76	0.678	0.846	1.044	1.293	1.665	1.992	2.376	2.642	3.201	3.423
77	0.678	0.846	1.043	1.293	1.665	1.991	2.376	2.641	3.199	3.421
78	0.678	0.846	1.043	1.292	1.665	1.991	2.375	2.640	3.198	3.420
79	0.678	0.846	1.043	1.292	1.664	1.990	2.374	2.640	3.197	3.418
80	0.678	0.846	1.043	1.292	1.664	1.990	2.374	2.639	3.195	3.416
81	0.678	0.846	1.043	1.292	1.664	1.990	2.373	2.638	3.194	3.415
82	0.677	0.846	1.043	1.292	1.664	1.989	2.373	2.637	3.193	3.413
83	0.677	0.846	1.043	1.292	1.663	1.989	2.372	2.636	3.191	3.412
84	0.677	0.846	1.043	1.292	1.663	1.989	2.372	2.636	3.190	3.410
85	0.677	0.846	1.043	1.292	1.663	1.988	2.371	2.635	3.189	3.409
86	0.677	0.846	1.043	1.291	1.663	1.988	2.370	2.634	3.188	3.407
87	0.677	0.846	1.043	1.291	1.663	1.988	2.370	2.634	3.187	3.406
88	0.677	0.846	1.043	1.291	1.662	1.987	2.369	2.633	3.185	3.405
89	0.677	0.846	1.043	1.291	1.662	1.987	2.369	2.632	3.184	3.403
90	0.677	0.846	1.042	1.291	1.662	1.987	2.368	2.632	3.183	3.402
91	0.677	0.846	1.042	1.291	1.662	1.986	2.368	2.631	3.182	3.401
92	0.677	0.846	1.042	1.291	1.662	1.986	2.368	2.630	3.181	3.399
93	0.677	0.846	1.042	1.291	1.661	1.986	2.367	2.630	3.180	3.398
94	0.677	0.845	1.042	1.291	1.661	1.986	2.367	2.629	3.179	3.397
95	0.677	0.845	1.042	1.291	1.661	1.985	2.366	2.629	3.178	3.396
96	0.677	0.845	1.042	1.290	1.661	1.985	2.366	2.628	3.177	3.395
97	0.677	0.845	1.042	1.290	1.661	1.985	2.365	2.627	3.176	3.394
98	0.677	0.845	1.042	1.290	1.661	1.984	2.365	2.627	3.175	3.393
99	0.677	0.845	1.042	1.290	1.660	1.984	2.365	2.626	3.175	3.392
100	0.677	0.845	1.042	1.290	1.660	1.984	2.364	2.626	3.174	3.390
101	0.677	0.845	1.042	1.290	1.660	1.984	2.364	2.625	3.173	3.389
102	0.677	0.845	1.042	1.290	1.660	1.983	2.363	2.625	3.172	3.388
103	0.677	0.845	1.042	1.290	1.660	1.983	2.363	2.624	3.171	3.388
104	0.677	0.845	1.042	1.290	1.660	1.983	2.363	2.624	3.170	3.387
105	0.677	0.845	1.042	1.290	1.659	1.983	2.362	2.623	3.170	3.386

(*Continued*)

(Continued)

106	0.677	0.845	1.042	1.290	1.659	1.983	2.362	2.623	3.169	3.385
107	0.677	0.845	1.041	1.290	1.659	1.982	2.362	2.623	3.168	3.384
108	0.677	0.845	1.041	1.289	1.659	1.982	2.361	2.622	3.167	3.383
109	0.677	0.845	1.041	1.289	1.659	1.982	2.361	2.622	3.167	3.382
110	0.677	0.845	1.041	1.289	1.659	1.982	2.361	2.621	3.166	3.381
111	0.677	0.845	1.041	1.289	1.659	1.982	2.360	2.621	3.165	3.380
112	0.677	0.845	1.041	1.289	1.659	1.981	2.360	2.620	3.165	3.380
113	0.677	0.845	1.041	1.289	1.658	1.981	2.360	2.620	3.164	3.379
114	0.677	0.845	1.041	1.289	1.658	1.981	2.360	2.620	3.163	3.378
115	0.677	0.845	1.041	1.289	1.658	1.981	2.359	2.619	3.163	3.377
116	0.677	0.845	1.041	1.289	1.658	1.981	2.359	2.619	3.162	3.376
117	0.677	0.845	1.041	1.289	1.658	1.980	2.359	2.619	3.161	3.376
118	0.677	0.845	1.041	1.289	1.658	1.980	2.358	2.618	3.161	3.375
119	0.677	0.845	1.041	1.289	1.658	1.980	2.358	2.618	3.160	3.374
120	0.677	0.845	1.041	1.289	1.658	1.980	2.358	2.617	3.160	3.373
↓	↓	↓	↓	↓	↓	↓	↓	↓	↓	↓
∞	0.674	0.842	1.036	1.282	1.645	1.960	2.326	2.576	3.090	3.291

Examples:

- A DF = 28 with a t-statistic = 0.82 can be found between 0.683 and 0.855. This corresponds to a 2-tailed p-value of between 0.40 and 0.50. Extrapolating to 0.82 gives a 2-tailed p-value of 0.417.
- A DF = 28 with a t-statistic = 2.49 can be found between 2.467 and 2.763. This corresponds to a 2-tailed p-value of between 0.02 and 0.01. Extrapolating to 2.49 gives a 2-tailed p-value of 0.019.

Glossary

A priori A decision or thought made or conceived beforehand.

Absolute risk *Frequency* of an *event* occurring in relation to the total *population* at *risk* for the *event* over time. Also known as *incidence*.

Absolute risk difference (ARD or RD) The difference in the absolute risk in the group with an intervention/exposure and the absolute risk in the group without an intervention/exposure. Also known as *attributable risk* or *risk difference*.

Absolute risk increase (ARI) A positive difference in *absolute risk* in the group with an *exposure/intervention* compared to the group without an *exposure/intervention*.

Absolute risk reduction (ARR) A negative difference in *absolute risk* in the group with an *exposure/intervention* compared to the group without an *exposure/intervention*.

Accuracy Estimation of how close the observed measurements are to the "truth" (e.g., the actual *population* parameter). Accuracy is negatively affected by *systematic errors* or *bias*.

Adjusted effect estimate A *measure of association* that accounts for the impact potential *confounders* may have on the estimate.

Allocation concealment Methods used in *randomized controlled trials* to guard or conceal the randomization sequence from the study personnel responsible for randomizing the patients as they are enrolled in the study.

"Alpha" (α) Predetermined cutoff value used to determine the statistical threshold for significance. It indicates the level for which researchers are willing to accept a false positive or reject the null hypothesis when it should not be rejected (*type I error*). Also known as the *significance level*.

Alternative hypothesis When a *null hypothesis* is rejected there must be another, an alternative hypothesis that explains the observed outcome. A hypothesis against which the null hypothesis is tested. An assumption that the observed data represent some real effect, beyond chance or other *systematic errors*. Sometimes expressed as H_A or H_1. Also known as the *test hypothesis*.

Analysis of variance (ANOVA) A statistical test typically used to determine the extent to which three or more group means in a sample are statistically significantly different from each other.

Analytical study A type of study that aims to quantify relationships between two or more variables by including a *control group* or *comparison group*.

Antecedent-consequent bias A type of bias in cross-sectional and case-control studies that occurs when it is incorrectly determined that an exposure preceded the occurrence of an

Statistics for Dental Clinicians, First Edition. Michael Glick, Alonso Carrasco-Labra, and Olivia Urquhart.
© 2024 John Wiley & Sons, Inc. Published 2024 by John Wiley & Sons, Inc.

outcome, or that an outcome preceded the occurrence of an exposure. Also known as *reverse causation* or *temporality bias*.

Applicability The extent to which study results can be generalized or extrapolated to other contexts, for example, a local clinical practice. Also known as *external validity* or *generalizability*.

Association The dependence of one *variable* on another variable or the relationship between two variables or when two *variables* are related. The direction of an association is symbolized by either a positive (+) or a negative (−) sign.

As-treated analysis A method to analyze data from a randomized controlled trial where study participants are included in the study group in which the intervention was received, regardless of whether they were randomized to receive that intervention.

Attributable risk See *absolute risk difference*.

Attrition bias A type of *selection bias* that occurs when the study participants that leave a study before it ends (loss to follow-up, missing participant data) are systematically different (the loss is related to the exposure or outcome) than those that remain in the study for the entirety of the follow-up period.

b A value for the slope in a correlation or a straight line.

Backdoor pathway In a *directed acyclic graph* (DAG), backdoor pathways are every possible alternative pathway that connect the *exposure* with the *outcome* that are not part of the direct pathway from the exposure of interest to the outcome. These pathways are sometimes also called confounding pathways.

Background risk The *absolute risk* among individuals not exposed to a risk factor or intervention. Also known as *baseline risk*.

Baseline risk See *background risk*.

Berkson's bias A type of *bias* that can occur in a *case-control study* when the *exposure* of interest results in individuals developing a medical issue that subsequently makes them seek health care, and therefore the *frequency* of the exposure among *controls* will be misleadingly high. This spuriously high frequency of exposure among controls can bias the *association*, obliterate it or even reverse its direction. Also known as *hospital patient bias*.

"Beta" (β) In hypothesis testing and in *sample size* estimations, a predetermined cutoff value indicating the level researchers are willing to accept a false negative or not rejecting the *null hypothesis* when the null hypothesis is "false"- making a *type II error*.
In regression, standardized coefficient used in regression analyses and studies of correlation (see *regression coefficient*).

Between-study variance In the context of a *meta-analysis*, differences in effects between studies beyond *random error*. It can be quantified numerically (typically abbreviated as the square of the Greek letter "τ" (tau)—τ^2). Also known as *heterogeneity*.

Bias Deviation of results or inferences from the truth due to limitations in the study design, or in the process of collection, analysis, interpretation, publication, or review of data. Biases can lead to systematic differences (as opposed to *random error*) from the "truth". Also known as *systematic error*.

Binary variable A *categorical variable* that can only take two possible values. For example, having or not having an event, or a 0 or a 1 value. Also known as *dichotomous variable*.

Biostatistics Application of statistical concepts and techniques to topics in biology, including the medical sciences.

Bivariate random effects model One of two preferred *meta-analysis* models for pooling diagnostic test accuracy data.

Blinding Methods used in analytical studies to mask study participants, research personnel, and clinician investigators from learning who were exposed and unexposed to a factor (e.g., *risk factor*) or an *intervention.*

Block randomization A method to randomly allocate study participants to study arms, in which blocks of equal size (an equal number of spots for each study arm) are associated with a random sequence. This method can avoid the potential issue of imbalance in the numbers of people assigned to each *study arm* that can occur when simple *randomization* alone is used to allocate study participants to study arms.

Cases Individuals in a study with the *outcome* of interest

Case-control study An observational study of persons with a disease of interest and a *control* without the disease of interest to assess the relationship between the presence of an attribute in the past, for example, a *risk factor* that could have explained the occurrence of the disease.

Categorical variable A *variable* with values that describe a "quality" or "characteristic" of a data unit, like "what type" or "which category or group" and tend to be represented by a non-numeric value. Also known as *qualitative variable.*

Causal inference A discipline of research that aims to disentangle connections between exposures and outcomes, including different relationships among them, for the purpose of predicting an exposure-outcome association or relationship.

Censoring In the context of survival analysis, study participants that were lost to follow-up, withdrew from the study, or did not experience the event of interest at the end of the study follow-up period.

Central limit theorem (CLT) The occurrence where independent *random variables*, when added, take on the shape of a *normal distribution* regardless of the shape (e.g., skewed distribution) of the population distribution when the *sample size* (n) is sufficiently large (~>30).

Central tendency A single descriptive summary of a data set that denotes the central or middle position within the data set. The three most common measures of central tendency are the *mean*, the *median*, and the *mode.*

Certainty of the evidence "In the context of a systematic review, the ratings of the certainty of evidence reflect the extent of our confidence that the estimates of the effect are close to the truth. In the context of making recommendations, the certainty ratings reflect the extent of our confidence that the estimates of an effect are adequate to support a particular decision or recommendation."[1] Also referred to as *quality of the evidence.*

Clinical practice guideline A document containing recommendations or options to aid in clinical decision making in areas of prevention, diagnosis, or treatment of a disease or condition. An evidence-based clinical practice guideline should be informed by systematic review(s) summarizing the underpinning evidence, which should be directly linked to the recommendations or options.

Clinical significance A magnitude of an effect that is relevant to patients, clinicians, or policymakers that warrants a change in practice or adopting a course of action.

---

1 Hulcratz M, Rind D, Akl EA, et al. The GRADE Working Group clarifies the construct of certainty of evidence. *J Clinical Epidemiol.* 2017;87: 4–13.

Clinical threshold Threshold defined as *clinically significant* (e.g., *minimal important difference*). In diagnostic test accuracy studies, the critical probability of making a diagnosis that assists a clinician in making appropriate treatment decisions or further workup or testing.

Clinical trial A prospective *experimental study* that compares the effect of one or more interventions against a *control group* or *comparison group* in human subjects.

Clinician-reported outcome Type of outcome with a construct that may or may not be a clinical parameter assessed or rated by a health care professional.

Cluster randomized controlled trial A *randomized controlled trial* where clusters or groups are randomized to the study arms. The unit of *randomization* is not an individual but rather a group like a school, hospital, or household.

Cluster sampling A sampling method where eligible individuals for a study naturally cluster in discrete geographic or organizational units. These clusters can be municipalities, hospitals, schools, or classes and become the unit of sampling from which investigators can draw a simple random sample.

Cochran's Q test In the context of a *meta-analysis*, a statistical test to assess the possible presence or absence of statistical *heterogeneity* (*between-study variance*).

Coefficient of determination A number describing the proportion of the *variance* in the dependent variable that is accounted for by the *independent variable*, under the assumption of a linear relationship. Mathematically it is the square of the *correlation coefficient* and is denoted by r^2 (when used in simple regression) or R^2 (when used in the context of multiple regression).

Cohen's kappa (κ) or chance-corrected agreement A statistic used to measure the level of agreement, typically between two observers (*inter-rater reliability*) who classify items into mutually exclusive categories. This statistic can provide a value that reflects the extent to which two raters achieve agreement beyond the level expected by chance alone (50%). The values of a Cohen's kappa range between 0% and 100%, with values around 75% being considered excellent agreement.

Cohort Group of individuals who share similar attributes.

Cohort study *Observational study* in which a group of individuals are followed over time to assess if there are differences in outcomes between individuals in the cohort that were exposed or not exposed to a potential *risk factor.*

Collinearity A linear *correlation* (two independent variables that correlate with each other), in regression modeling, where the inclusion of both variables in the model could be redundant and lead to issues when interpreting the *regression coefficients.*

Combined effect estimate A single estimate derived from a *meta-analysis* reflecting the weighted average of the results from two or more primary studies, often represented with a diamond-like symbol in a *forest plot*. Also known as *pooled effect estimate and summary effect estimate.*

Comparator In *analytical studies*, the group that did not receive the *intervention* (therapeutic or new diagnostic test) or the nonexposed group that is compared with the exposed group. In *case-control studies*, although also an analytical study, the group without the *outcome* or disease of interest (*controls*). Also known as *reference group or control group.*

Composite outcome The combination of two or more *outcomes* into a single outcome.

Comparative effectiveness research A type of research in which the benefits and harms of two or more preventive, diagnostic, or treatment strategies are compared through the generation and synthesis of evidence.

Concurrent cohort study A *cohort study* where the investigators measure potential *risk factors* (i.e., *exposures*) at the beginning of the study and collect data on *outcomes* over time as the study is conducted. Also known as *prospective cohort study.*

Confidence coefficient The percentage of all possible *samples* that can be expected to include the true population *parameter*. A 95% confidence coefficient implies that 95% of *confidence intervals* would include the true population parameter. Also known as *confidence level*.

Confidence interval A range of values reflecting how much uncertainty there is with the observed data from a trial, an experiment, a survey, or the likes in relation to the true value in the *population* of interest. It assumes that the underlying methods to conduct and analyze a study are appropriate and free from *bias*. A confidence interval will contain the true population *parameter* with a frequency equivalent to the magnitude of its *confidence coefficient* (e.g., 95%).

Confidence level See *confidence coefficient*.

Confounder An *independent variable* that has a systematic influence on both the independent (*exposure*) and the *dependent (outcome) variable*, causing a spurious association, but does not lie in the causative pathway. Also known as *confounding variable*.

Confounding An issue affecting the validity of analytical studies, and represents the inability to control or adjust for *confounders* that can distort the potential exposure-outcome association under investigation.

Confounding by indication When some variable influences the reason why an intervention may be clinically indicated for some individuals and not others (e.g., individuals with a severe form of a disease may be more likely to receive a certain drug compared to individuals with a less severe form of the disease) and the outcome of interest, in turn, distorts the association being assessed.

Confounding variable See *confounder*.

Conflict of interest A special type of *bias* that emerges when the judgment of the researchers regarding their primary interest—conducting and reporting sound clinical research—is influenced by a second competing interest such as career promotion, financial gain, or prestige.

Construct The aspect/attribute that an instrument (e.g., a health questionnaire) aims to measure.

Construct validity Denotes that a questionnaire or instrument (e.g., a patient-reported outcome measure) provides valid results (see *validity*). It allows drawing accurate conclusions about the *construct* of interest or health status.

Content validity Denotes that an instrument or questionnaire appropriately covers all aspects of the *construct*.

Continuous variable A numeric *variable* that can take any number of countless values between a certain set of real numbers (e.g., age, height).

Control group See *comparator*.

Convenience sampling *Sampling* method where the selection of individuals is based solely on their availability or willingness to participate in the study.

Correlation The extent to which a change in the value of one (can also be more than one), variable—the *independent variable*(s)—results in a corresponding—by a fixed amount—change on a second variable—the *dependent variable*.

Correlation coefficient A measure of association that provides information about whether a relationship exists between two or more variables and describes the strength and direction of such a relationship. One of the more common correlation coefficients is the *Pearson correlation* (*r*).

Counterfactual framework Theoretical concept in which the occurrence of outcomes is compared in an individual exposed to a risk or protective factor to a fictitious scenario (counter to the facts) where the same individual under the exact same conditions (e.g., same point in time, same environment, etc.) is not exposed to the risk or protective factor.

Cox proportional hazard model A regression approach to determine the association between a time-to-event outcome of interest and one (univariable) or more covariates or predictors (multivariable).

Cross-sectional study An *observational study* where data are collected from a *population* at a single point in time. Both *exposures* and *outcomes* are measured simultaneously, disregarding their temporality (i.e., whether the exposure occurred before the outcome or whether the outcome occurred before the exposure).

Crude effect estimate A *measure of association* estimate that has not been adjusted for potential *confounders*.

Cumulative incidence The number of new cases of disease as a proportion of the *population* without the disease at baseline. Also known as incidence proportion.

Cumulative probability In *survival analysis*, the product of the probability of survival from the beginning of an interval in a *Kaplan–Meier survival curve* to the end of the interval, which is the same time point as the beginning of the next interval.

Dependent variable The variable that changes as a result of changes in an *independent variable*. It's the outcome of interest and it "depends" on the independent variable(s). The dependent variable is often represented on the y-axis of a graph. These variables can also be referred to as *outcome*, response, or *predicted variable*.

Descriptive statistics Measures that allow for the summarization of key features of a *sample* from a *population*, often reported in tables and graphs. Examples of descriptive statistics (here statistics means data collected with statistical methods) include measures of *central tendency* (*mean*, *median*, or *mode*), measures of variability (e.g., *standard deviation*, range, variance), distributions of the data, and *confidence intervals*.

Descriptive study A type of study that aims to summarize the *distribution* of *variables* without trying to explain the relationship between variables (e.g., a study depicting a phenomenon, *such as*, the frequency of a disease or condition in a *population*).

Detection bias A type of information bias that occurs when the ascertainment or measurement of the disease or outcome of interest is systematically different between exposed and unexposed groups.

Determinant A factor causally responsible for a modification in the *risk* of experiencing an *outcome*, such as acquiring a disease or condition. *Risk factors* are identified by examining determinants that influence the occurrence of new cases of disease. It is not the same as a *prognostic factor*. Also known as *risk factor*.

Dichotomous variable See *binary variable*.

Differential misclassification bias A type of information bias that occurs when the frequency of incorrect classification of an exposure or outcome is dependent on the outcome or exposure status of the individual, respectively results in a distortion of the research findings.

Direct effect estimate An effect estimate derived from an analytical study.

Directed acyclic graphs (DAGs) A diagram that represents an underpinning causal theory. This diagram provides a hypothetical explanation of how the *exposure* of interest affects the *outcome* and other variables that may influence or be affected by the exposure and outcome. The resulting causal model is essential to determine study participants' selection and identify variables (e.g., *confounding variables*) that should be measured and accounted for later in the statistical analysis.

Discrete variable A numeric *variable* that can take any number of countable values from a set of distinct whole values but cannot take the value of a fraction between one value and the next closest value (e.g., number of admissions to a hospital, number of people who have periodontal disease).

Distribution A representation of all possible values (or intervals) of scores, and the frequency (how often) each score occurs. In an example of weight, a specific weight in a sample is a value that can be represented as a score in a distribution. The frequency is how often a specific weight is observed. A distribution is often depicted as a graph, e.g., a normal curve depicting a normal distribution with the score on the x-axis and the frequency on the y-axis or as a table.

Effect A difference between what was observed or measured and the true population *parameter*. An effect is the result, for example, of applying an *intervention*, treatment, a public health policy, the impact of a disease outbreak, or a genetic mutation.

Effect estimate A measure of the magnitude of an *association* between *exposure/intervention* and *outcomes* derived from observed data.

Effectiveness Effect of an *intervention* (e.g., a treatment) under real-world conditions.

Effect modification/effect modifier The *association* between an *exposure* and an *outcome* of interest affected or modified by a third variable—the modifier. Exploring effect modification allows for the identification of subgroups or patient groups that would benefit more or less from an *intervention*, improving preventive or therapeutic interventions. Also known as *subgroup effect,* or *interaction*.

Effect size A standardized measure without units, commonly used to compare the magnitude of effects between different *interventions* or *exposures*.

Efficacy Beneficial and harmful effects or performance of a treatment compared to a *control group* under ideal and controlled situations and all study participants adhere to the allocated treatment protocol.

Epidemiology The study of the distribution and determinants of disease and health in human populations.

Etiological study A study that aims to quantitatively determine the causal relationship between *exposures* (*risk factors*) and an *outcome* (condition or disease) of interest.

Event Something that could possibly occur for which one wants to know the chance of it occurring. For example, the presence of caries lesions can be an event for the *outcome* "presence or absence of caries lesions". Rolling a 3 on a die can be an event for the possible outcomes of rolling a die. "Getting a head" can be an event for the possible outcomes of flipping a coin.

Event rate See *risk*.

Exchangeability of baseline risks When the expected *baseline risks* of experiencing the *outcome* are the same between groups in an analytical study (i.e., both group 1 and 2 have a baseline risk of 30%). A *measure of association* computed under this scenario is considered an unconfounded *association*.

Experimental study A study in which the investigator deliberately chooses which study participants receive the *intervention*(s) of interest and which study participants receive the control intervention (e.g., active intervention, *placebo*, or no *intervention*).

External validity See *applicability*.

Exposure The presence of a factor, a characteristic, or any external agent that could cause, explain, or predict an *outcome*.

F-statistic A ratio of the *variance* between groups, which represent the dispersion across the entire dataset to the variance within the group under comparison. In an *ANOVA test*, a large F-statistic (associated with a small *p-value*) suggests that the differences among the group means are statistically significant. In regression analysis, the F-statistic is used to determine the overall statistical significance of the model, with a large F-statistic (associated with a small *p-value*) indicates that the model predicts the *dependent variable* significantly better than using the mean of the dependent variable.

Face validity Attribute of a question or a survey instrument, that represent the experience by patients or their caregivers or parents who are aware of what the disease is about and what it means for their lives, for a condition of interest.

Factor Another name for *variable*.

Failure In the context of *survival analysis*, an indication that an *event* of interest has occurred in an individual.

False negative rate (FNR) The *probability* of a negative test result in a person with the disease, (can be represented by 1 − *sensitivity*).

False positive rate (FPR) The *probability* of a positive test result in a person without the disease, (can be represented by 1 − *specificity*).

Fixed effect meta-analysis A type of model in the context of a *meta-analysis* that assumes all of the studies are estimating the same (treatment) *effect* or equal effect, and any difference observed is the result of *random error*.

Follow-up Observation of a variable such as an *outcome* of interest over a specific period of time to determine the extent and magnitude of a change in such a *variable* or outcome.

Forest plot A specific graphical depiction of data inputs and results of a *meta-analysis*

Frequency The number of times something occurs over a certain period of time.

Generalizability See applicability and external validity.

Generic inverse-variance method A method for weighting studies in a *meta-analysis* derived by taking the inverse of the variance of a given study.

Goodness-of-fit test In the context of regression modeling, a test that quantifies how well the model fits the observed data.

Gold standard A test or measurement that is perceived to be the best available/most accurate way to diagnose a disease or to assess the presence of an *outcome*.

Hazard The slope of a *survival curve* that represents how rapidly subjects are experiencing the *event* of interest at any point in time. A hazard rate is also defined as the *risk* of having an event of interest at a particular point in time. It is the opposite of the *survival rate*. Also known as *hazard rate*.

Hazard rate See *hazard*.

Hazard ratio A ratio of *hazard rates*. It is a measure of the *effect* of two *interventions* (or *prognostic factors*) on an *event* of interest, comparing the *risk* of an event in one group with the risk of the event in the *comparison group* at any time during the entire study period.

Heterogeneity See between-study variance.

Hierarchical summary receiver operating curve (ROC) model One of two preferred *meta-analysis* models for pooling diagnostic test accuracy data.

Hospital patient bias See *Berkson's bias*,

Hypothesis testing A statistical method that allows comparing a p-value against a prespecified level of significance ("*alpha*" α) to determine whether a *test hypothesis* (e.g., null) should be rejected.

I^2 ("I square") In the context of a *meta-analysis*, a measure (statistic) quantifying the extent of *heterogeneity* across studies. It ranges from 0% to 100%, where 0% means that there may be no heterogeneity, and 100% is the highest level of heterogeneity.

Incidence A measure of the number of new cases of disease or injury that develop in a *population* over a particular time period.

Incidence proportion See *cumulative incidence*.

Incidence rate The number of new cases of disease as a proportion of the *risk* free time individuals contribute to the study (person-time at risk).

Incidence density ratio A *measure of association* estimated in cohort studies representing the ratio of the *incidence rate* in an exposed group and the incidence rate in an unexposed group. Also known as *rate ratio*.

Incident cases Individuals who recently developed the *outcome* of interest within the observation period.

Independent variable The *variable* being changed, controlled, or manipulated in an *experimental study* to explore its effects. It's called "independent" because it is assumed that it is not influenced by any other *variables* in the study. The independent variable is often represented on the x-axis of a graph. These variables can also be referred to as predictors, exposures, covariates, or explanatory variables.

Index test A diagnostic test of interest that is evaluated against a reference test (a *gold standard*) in a study of diagnostic test accuracy.

Indirect effect estimate An *effect estimate* describing the comparison of two *interventions* or *exposures* that have not been directly compared in a study.

Inferential statistics Methods for using data from a *sample* to make generalizations or draw conclusions about a population of interest.

Information bias A group of biases that can affect the *validity* of a study when investigators fail to appropriately measure, classify or interpret data related to *exposures* and *outcomes*. See *detection bias, misclassification bias, nondifferential misclassification bias, observer bias, recall bias*.

Intention-to-treat analysis A method to analyze data from a *randomized controlled trial* where study participants are included in the study group they were initially randomized, regardless of whether they actually received the intervention intended for that group.

Interval scale A type of numeric measurement where the values can fall below 0 (e.g., temperature). These scales do not have a "true" 0, which means that measuring 0 does not imply absence of the attribute.

Interaction term An expression included in a regression model representing the product of a potential *effect modifier* and exposure of interest.

Internal consistency The extent to which the items or questions in an instrument relate to each other and reflect the same *construct*. Cronbach's alpha is typically used to measure internal consistency.

Internal validity Degree of confidence that the study results represent the truth in the population under evaluation and are not distorted by other factors or variables such as *bias* and *confounding*.

Inter-rater reliability A measure of *reliability* which reflects the degree of agreement between two or more observers.

Interval estimate Representation of the *precision* of a point estimate and indicates how much the sample statistic differs from the *population mean* (e.g., *confidence interval*).

Intervention Any type of education, training, behavioral modification, surgical procedure, pharmacological agent, public health program, or accommodation for the provision of care received by participants in a clinical trial.

Intra-rater reliability A measure of *reliability* which considers the degree of agreement between the same observer at two different time points. It assumes that the trait assessed by the rater has not changed between the assessments.

Kaplan–Meier survival curve A *survival curve* that is depicted using the Kaplan–Meier method to estimate survival time.

Likelihood ratio (LR) The likelihood of a positive test result (for a positive likelihood ratio) or a negative test result (for a negative likelihood ratio) in a patient with a disease of interest as a ratio to the likelihood of the same test result in a patient without the disease of interest.

Likert scale Response scale that often includes 7 or 5 categories to determine a responder's level of agreement with a statement. For example: (1) not at all important, (2) low importance, (3) slightly important, (4) neutral, (5) moderately important, (6) very important, and (7) extremely important.

Linear regression A regression model describing the relationship between one or more *independent variables* and a *continuous dependent variable*.

Logistic regression A regression model describing the relationship between one or more *independent variables* and a *categorical dependent variable*.

Log-rank test A statistical test to compare two or more *survival curves*; emphasizes distances between the curves at the end of the curve (later in the study).

Magnitude Another word for size.

Mantel–Haenszel method A method to calculate *weights* in a *meta-analysis* when data are sparse (events are rare or studies are small).

Margin of error The range of values above or below the point estimate within a confidence interval.

Matching A strategy to deal with *confounding* in the design phase of a study where investigators select cases and controls (*case-control study*) or exposed and unexposed (*cohort study*) individuals with similar attributes or levels of a confounding variable.

Mean The average of all numbers within a dataset.

Mean difference (MD) A *measure of association* expressed as the difference between two *means* measured with the same scale. When the MD equals zero, there is no difference between the means of two groups.

Measures of association A value expressing the strength or magnitude of an *association* or a treatment effect between two groups of interest. (e.g., *risk ratio, odds ratio, hazard ratio,* differences in *means,* proportions, *risks,* rates, *correlation,* and *regression coefficients*).

Measurement bias Distortion in the study results due to dissimilar management (performance) of groups under comparison as a study is conducted or a systematic difference in the procedures used to determine (measure) the outcomes. Blinding is frequently used to minimize the impact of performance and measurement bias. Also known as *performance bias.*

Measurement scales See *interval scale, nominal scale, ordinal scale,* and *ratio scale.*

Median A point that divides a score into two with half the scores above and half the scores below the point.

Median survival time The time elapsed for which 50% of individuals in a *survival analysis* have survived.

Meta-analysis A statistical technique that synthesizes and combines the results from two or more studies to assess the dispersion of effects, distinguish between real and spurious dispersions, and provide a *summary effect* of all included studies.

Meta-regression An extension of a classic *meta-analysis* in which regression models are used to test and account for potential *subgroup effects* across studies. The *independent variables* are attributes of the study that could affect the *dependent variable*—the *pooled effect estimate.*

Methodological quality The extent to which study authors conducted their research to the highest possible methodological standards.

Metric A set of numbers that give information about a particular process or activity.

Minimal import difference The smallest within-person change in the score of an *outcome* (beneficial or harmful) that people perceive as important.

Misclassification bias A type of *information bias* where the *exposure* and/or *outcome* status of study participants is categorized incorrectly.

Mixed effect estimate An effect estimate derived from a *network meta-analysis* that is a combination of the *direct* and *indirect effect estimates*. Also known as *network effect estimate.*

Mode The most frequent score in a set of data.

Multiple linear regression A regression model describing the relationship between a continuous dependent variable and more than one independent variable. Also known as *multivariable linear regression.*

Multiple logistic regression A *logistic regression* model describing the relationship between a *categorical dependent variable* and more than one *independent variable*. Also known as *multivariable logistic regression.*

Multiple regression A regression model describing the relationship between one or more independent variables and a categorical dependent variable. Also known as *multivariable regression.*

Multivariable regression See *multiple regression.*

Multivariable linear regression See *multiple linear regression.*

Multivariable logistic regression See *multiple logistic regression.*

Multistage sampling A sampling method where sampling occurs in stages, where the sampling unit or the group being sampled becomes smaller and smaller at each stage. Often implemented using a combination of sampling strategies.

Naïve per-protocol analysis A method to analyze data from a *randomized controlled trial* where only study participants who adhere to the study arm they were allocated to are included in the data analysis.

Negative likelihood ratio (LR−) The odds of a disease in a person with a disease and a negative test result as a ratio of the odds of a person without the disease and a negative test result.

Negative predictive value (NPV) The chance (*probability*) of a person with a negative test result not having the disease of interest; the percentage of all true negative test results among all negative test results—true negative/(true negative + false negative).

Network effect estimate See *mixed effect estimate.*

Network meta-analysis A type of *meta-analysis* that facilitates the comparison of three or more *effects* simultaneously, by combining evidence from *interventions* directly compared in studies and evidence from interventions not directly compared in studies (*indirect effect estimate*).

Neyman bias A type of selection bias that occurs when the sampling process facilitates the inclusion of a disproportionally high percentage of individuals with the *outcome* of interest or *cases* with long disease duration over other individuals with a more severe progression and shorter duration, which would prevent or minimize their chances of being sampled. Also known as *prevalence-incidence bias.*

Nominal scale A measurement that can take a value that is not able to be organized in a logical sequence (e.g., marital status—married, single, widowed, divorced/separated).

Nonconcurrent cohort study A type of cohort study in which investigators take advantage of data already available and collected in the past. These data are obtained from cohorts that were formed in the past—retrospective or historical cohorts. In most situations, these data were collected for purposes other than the study at hand; these data precede or are nonconcurrent with the conduct of the study. Also known as *retrospective cohort study.*

Nondifferential misclassification bias A type of *information bias* that occurs when the *frequency* of the incorrect classification of an exposure or outcome is independent from the individual's outcome or exposure status respectively, which results in a distortion of the research findings.

Nonparticipation bias A type of *selection bias* that occurs when important differences in the *exposure* and subsequent outcome exist between eligible individuals that respond to a survey, questionnaire, or invitation to be part of a study and those who decline the invitation.

Nonprobabilistic sampling Sampling methods not using probabilities but convenience or subjective criteria to identify a study sample.

Nonresponse bias A type of *selection bias* that occurs when important differences in the exposure exist between eligible individuals that respond to a survey, questionnaire, or invitation to be part of a study and those who ignore the invitation.

Normal distribution A normal distribution includes 100% of all possible scores where 50% of the scores are above the mean and 50% of the scores are below the mean, and 1 standard deviation surrounding the mean includes approximately 68% of all possible scores; 2 standard deviations surrounding the mean include a tad more than 95% of all possible scores; and 3 standard deviations surrounding the mean include more than 99% of all possible scores. The normal distribution is a continuous distribution, and therefore the scores for a normally distributed variable can take on any one of a countless number of possible values. The graphic depiction of a normal distribution is often referred to as a bell-shaped curve or the Gaussian curve.

Normalize The process of recasting different variables so they can be viewed on the same scale. This process allows comparison of scores between different types of variables. Also known as *standardize*.

Null hypothesis (H_0) The primary hypothesis to be tested in *hypothesis testing*. It is based on an assumption that two or more population distributions are not different, or that there is no association between two or more sets of variables.

Number needed to treat for benefit (NNTB) The number of individuals in the intervention group who would need to be treated for one additional person to experience a beneficial or favorable outcome.

Number needed to treat for harm (NNTH) The number of individuals in the intervention group who need to be treated for one additional person to avoid a harmful or unfavorable outcome.

Numeric variable A variable that has values that describe a measurable quantity as a number, like "how many" or "how much." Also known as *quantitative variable*.

Observational study Type of study where investigators observe characteristics in a sample or *population* and take measurements. This differ from other study designs, for example, experimental designs where an investigator actively assigns an intervention of interest.

Observer bias A type of *information bias* that ensues when investigators are aware of the disease status or outcome of interest and ask leading questions so that participants' responses confirm the investigators' hypothesis.

Odds The likelihood of an event occurring as a *proportion* of the event not occurring.

Odds ratio A *measure of association* between an exposed and unexposed group, or a group receiving and not receiving an *intervention*. The quotient of the *odds* (likelihood) of an *event* occurring given a particular *exposure*/intervention divided by the odds of the event not occurring in the absence of that exposure/intervention.

Oral-health-related quality of life (OHRQL) A type of *patient-reported outcome measure* reflecting a patient's subjective assessment of how personal oral health-related matters may affect their quality of life.

Ordinal scale A measurement that can take a value that can be logically ordered or ranked, but the distance between the categories is unknown (e.g., size of a car—subcompact, compact, midsize, or large).

Ordinary least squares (OLS) method A technique to derive *regression coefficients* in *linear regression*. The difference in the actual data points from a sample and the estimated fitted values (i.e., the line of best fit) is called the sample residuals. Ordinary least squares method is a way of estimating regression coefficients to minimize these sample residuals or the distance between the estimated line of best fit and the sample data.

Outcome Construct or *variable* of interest in a research study that is speculated to be caused by another variable, for example, a clinical intervention or an exposure. The word *effect* is sometimes used interchangeably.

Outcome measure Explicit definition of how an *outcome* of interest will be assessed and recorded in participants involved in a clinical study. Outcome measures can be *continuous* (e.g., oral health-related quality of life measured using the OHIP-14 questionnaire, mouth opening in millimeters, pain measured using a visual analog scale in centimeters, clinical attachment level in millimeters), *ordinal* (e.g., low, moderate, high income; pain intensity measured as no pain, mild, moderate, severe, extreme; any Likert scale), or *categorical* (e.g., presence or absence of a caries lesion, pulp necrosis, dental implant failure).

Overall effect estimate See *pooled effect estimate.*

Overmatching Denotes when matching is implemented in the design stage of a study, but the potential *confounding variable* that is used to match the groups is not actually a *confounder.* If the variable remains associated with the *exposure* while it is not related to the outcome (failing to meet the criteria for a confounder), the study *power* would be reduced by making *cases* and controls more similar.

P-value A *probability* (continuous measure) representing the compatibility (p close to 1.0 suggests high compatibility; p close to 0 suggests low compatibility) of the observed data with a prespecified statistical model, which assumes that the null hypothesis is true. The use of the letter "p" stands for probability.

Pairwise meta-analysis A type of meta-analysis where the effect estimate of interest, for example, a relative risk comparing the *frequency* of outcomes between two groups, such as two arms of a *clinical trial*, two exposure groups from an *observational study*, is examined for a single comparison.

Patient-important outcomes *Outcomes* that patients value or care about with regards to their health status, to distinguish them from surrogate outcomes, physiological measures, or clinical indicators that a clinician may consider important.

Patient-reported outcome measures Indices, instruments, tools, or questionnaires developed to measure a patient-reported outcome, which provide critical information about a person's experience or perspective regarding their health state. These types of outcomes are directly informed by the person or patient, without interpretation of the response by a third party (e.g., clinician, caregiver). Also referred to as a person-reported outcome measure.

Parallel randomized controlled trial A *randomized controlled trial* where individual study *participants* are randomized to two or more study arms.

Parameter A value that describes some aspect of a *population.* May also be referred to as population parameter. Parameters are denoted with Greek letters, e.g. μ (mu) = population mean; σ (sigma) = population standard deviation.

Pearson product-moment correlation coefficient (r) Also referred to as the *Pearson correlation coefficient* or *Pearson's r*, is one of the most common measures of association used in science to examine linear relationships between *continuous variables.*

Performance bias See *measurement bias.*

Performance-based outcome An *outcome* that is measured by a health care professional while the patient performs a task or set of tasks as instructed by a health care professional.

Period prevalence The number of cases of a disease or condition over a time interval (e.g., the prevalence of COVID-19 in the United States during 2020).

Person-time The amount of disease-free time that an individual contributes to a study from baseline to either 1) the time point when the *outcome* of interest occurred,

2) the time point when the study ends and the outcome did not yet occur (i.e., *censored*), or 3) the time point when a person is considered lost to follow-up.

Peto's method A method to calculate weights in a *fixed effect meta-analysis* model combining *odds ratios*.

Peto's test A statistical test to compare two or more *survival curves*; emphasizes distances between the curves at the beginning of the curve (early on in the study)

Placebo An inactive medication or procedure intended to give study participants in a *clinical trial* the appearance of receiving the *intervention* of interest.

Pretest probability The probability of disease before any examination or testing. Also known as *prior probability*.

Point estimate Estimate of a *statistic* from a *sample* for a *population parameter*.

Point prevalence The number of cases of a disease or condition at a single point in time (e.g., the prevalence of COVID-19 in the United States on March 19, 2020).

Pooled effect estimate See *combined effect estimate*.

Positive likelihood ratio The odds of disease in a person with a disease and a positive test result as a ratio of the odds of a person without the disease and a *positive test result*.

Positive predictive value (PPV) The chance (probability) of a person with a positive test having the disease; the percentage of all true positive test results among all positive test results—true positive/(true positive + false positive).

Posttest probability The probability of disease after clinical workup and testing. Also known as posterior probability.

Posterior probability See *posttest probability*.

Population A certain group of individuals or categories that represents all the members of interest, or all members of a group about which we want to draw a conclusion, or the whole group for which results are applicable.

Power The power of a test denotes the probability of detecting a difference when a difference does exist between the groups being compared; the capacity to correctly rejecting the *null hypothesis* when it should be rejected; $1-\beta$ equals statistical power.

Precision A function of replicability—how close to each other are replicated measurements. Precision reflects *random error*.

Predicted variable See *dependent variable*.

Prediction interval A range of values similar to a confidence interval in the sense that the uncertainty in the observed data from a trial, an experiment, a survey, or the likes in relation to the true value in the *population* of interest is accounted for. Prediction intervals also account for variability in individual data points and therefore represent the uncertainty around a prediction for an event that will occur in the future. Prediction intervals are wider than confidence intervals.

Predictor variable See *independent variable*.

Prevalence A measure of the number of cases of, for example, a disease in a population of interest at a specific time point as a proportion of the total number of individuals in the population.

Prevalence-incidence bias See *Neyman bias*.

Prevalence odds ratio An *odds ratio* computed in *cross-sectional studies* comparing the *prevalence* of disease between an exposed and unexposed group.

Prevalence ratio A *risk ratio* computed in *cross-sectional studies* comparing the *prevalence* of disease between an exposed and unexposed group.

Prevalent cases Individuals who already experienced the *outcome* of interest at some point in the past within the observation period.

Prior probability See *pretest probability*

Probability A measure of how likely it is that something will occur; the relative frequency of the occurrence of a particular event among all equally likely events. For example, the probability of throwing a "2" with a regular six-sided die is 1 out of 6 (getting a 1, 2, 3, 4, 5, or 6 are 6 equally likely events); the probability of getting a "head" when flipping a non-biased coin, is 1 out of 2 (getting a "head" or getting a "tail" are 2 equally likely events). A probability of 0 means that the event will never occur, while a probability of 1 means that an event will always occur. Any probability between 0 and 1 (can be expressed as a decimal number or as a percentage) means that the event will occur some part of the time. For example, a probability of 0.6, which can be expressed as a probability of 60%, means that an event will occur 6 times out of a possible 10 times where all 10 times being equally likely to occur.

Probabilistic sampling Methods of selecting a *sample* using *probability* theory. The key feature of this type of sampling is that any individual in the *population* of interest has the same chance of being selected for the study.

Prognostic balance An equal distribution of known and unknown *prognostic factors* among study arms.

Prognostic factor Factor responsible for experiencing a future health outcome in an individual who has been diagnosed with a particular disease or health condition. Prognostic factors are examined by following up people who already have a disease or condition of interest. It is not the same as a risk factor (see *risk factor*).

Prognostic study A study that aims to determine how prognostic factors affect the nature and frequency of the downstream consequences or outcomes associated with the disease, the condition, or the treatment.

Propensity score *Probability* for each individual to receive an *intervention* or treatment of interest given their specific level of *prognostic factors*.

Propensity-score adjustment Strategy to deal with confounding in the analysis phase of a study in which a propensity score is calculated for each individual and this information is included as a predictor in a multivariable regression model or used as a tool to choose matched pairs emulating a matching approach to adjusting for *confounding*. Also known as *propensity-score matching*.

Propensity-score matching See *propensity-score adjustment*.

Proportion A value derived by dividing the number of *events* by the total number of possible events. The events in the numerator are included in the denominator.

Proportional hazard assumption An assumption that the hazard rates in survival analysis always are proportional among two or more groups under comparison.

Prospective cohort study See *concurrent cohort study*.

Protective factor A factor that is expected to decrease the chance of an individual experiencing an undesirable outcome, such as acquiring a disease or condition.

Purposive sampling Sampling method that includes the identification of participants based on the study purpose or a set of subjective characteristics used as eligibility criteria.

Qualitative variable See *categorical variable*.

Quality of the evidence See *certainty of the evidence*.

Quantitative variable See *numeric variable*.

Quartile A statistical term that describes a division of observations into four defined intervals based on the values of the data and how they compare to the entire set of observations.

Random effects meta-analysis A type of model in the context of a *meta-analysis* that assumes the true effect from all studies are related but different. The *pooled effect* represents an average of effects across studies.

Random error Variation or discrepancy between a measure or observation and the true value in the population of interest due to the play of chance. Also known as random sampling error or variation, or sampling error.

Random sample Every member of a population has an equal chance of being selected into a sample or every member of a sample has an equal chance of being selected into a group.

Random sampling error See *random error*.

Random sampling variation See *random error*.

Random sequence In the context of a randomized controlled trial, a list of randomly generated numbers that indicates the allocation of participants to study arms.

Random variable A particular characteristic of an entity that can be measured (e.g. weight) or categorized (e.g. gender) that can assume different values purely by chance.

Randomization Allocation of study participants to intervention and comparison arms by chance. Also known as random allocation.

Randomized controlled trial (RCT) Type of clinical trial in which investigators are interested in the effect of an *intervention* or *exposure* administered intentionally, with participants randomly assigned to study arms under a controlled environment.

Rate Measure of how quickly something occurs.

Ratio A comparison of two quantities with the same units.

Ratio of means (ROM) A *measure of association* derived by comparing the *ratio* of two *means* the quotient of the mean in one group divided by the mean in another group.

Rate ratio See incidence density ratio.

Ratio scale A type of numeric measurement where the values cannot fall below 0 (e.g., body weight, height). These scales have a "true" 0, which means that measuring 0 implies absence of the attribute.

Recall bias A type of *information bias* that arises when study participants' disease status affects their likelihood of reporting an *exposure*.

Reference group See *comparator*.

Regression Statistical model that describes the relationship between the expected value of a *dependent variable* and one or more *independent variables* in the form of an equation that can be used to make inferences about the effect of an *intervention* or *exposure* on an *outcome*, as well as prognosis and prediction. See *linear regression*, *logistic regression*, *multiple or multivariable linear regression*, *multiple or multivariable logistic regression*, *multiple or multivariable regression*, simple logistic regression and *simple linear regression*.

Regression coefficient Values derived from fitting data with a regression model that represents estimates of population *parameters*. The values of regression coefficients describe the relationship between the *independent variables*(s) and *dependent variable*.

Relative risk (RR) A *measure of association* expressed as the quotient of the *absolute risk* of an *event*, such as disease, between exposed and unexposed groups, or participants receiving and not receiving an *intervention*. Also known as *prevalence ratio* and *risk ratio*.

Relative risk difference (RRD) The difference between the absolute risk in the exposed/ intervention group and the unexposed/control group as a proportion of the absolute risk in the unexposed/control group. When the risk in the exposed/intervention group is lower than the nonexposed/control group, the difference is called relative risk reduction (negative sign). When the risk in the exposed/intervention group is higher than the nonexposed/control group, the difference is called relative risk increase (positive sign).

Reliability Refers to the extent to which an instrument (e.g., a questionnaire) or a tool is able to provide consistent results or scores, free from measurement errors.

Reporting quality Comprehensiveness and appropriateness of the description of what was done, found, and concluded in a research study.

Results Any data collected when conducting a research study. A subset of these data is often reported in a scientific manuscript in the result section (e.g., population demographics, *risk* or *prognostic factors*, *events*, or measurement values of the *outcome* measures). Also known as study results.

Restriction A strategy to deal with *confounding* in the design phase of a study where the investigator utilizes the study eligibility criteria to exclude participants with the *confounding variable*. Also known as specification.

Retrospective cohort study See *nonconcurrent cohort study*.

Reverse causality See *antecedent-consequent bias*.

Risk The *probability* for an *event* to happen over a specified period. It could be a desirable or an undesirable *event*. Risk has neither a positive nor a negative connotation in statistics.

Risk difference (RD) See *absolute risk difference*.

Risk factor See *determinant*.

Risk of bias The extent to which the results of a research study are affected by *systematic error* or *bias*.

Risk ratio See *relative risk*.

Robust Robustness refers to the strength of a statistical model, a test, or a result from an analysis to assumptions, methodological decisions, and other study limitations.

Sample A representative subgroup selected from a *population*; a representative subset of a population.

Sample size Number of participants included in a study.

Sampling The process of identifying eligible subjects for a study. See *convenience sampling, nonprobabilistic sampling, purposive sampling, and snowball sampling*.

Sampling bias A type of *selection bias* that results when some individuals from the population of interest are more likely than other individuals to be enrolled in the study (nonrandom selection).

Sampling distribution The distribution of sample statistics computed for all possible *samples* of the same size taken from the same *population*. For *continuous variables*, we are interested in the sampling distribution of sample *means*, and for a *categorical variable* we are interested in the sampling distribution of sample proportions.

Sampling error See *random error*.

Scatterplot A graphical representation of the potential *association* between two *quantitative variables* of interest.

Selection bias A distortion in a *measure of association* or treatment effect arising from procedures to identify individuals to enter a study or to be included in the study analysis. See *Neyman's bias, nonparticipation bias, nonresponse bias*, and *sampling bias*.

Selective outcome reporting Type of bias that occurs when researchers deviate from the original protocol by omitting *outcomes* from the final report with the purpose of making the *intervention* look more favorable than if the entire efficacy and safety outcomes were disclosed.

Sensitivity The chance (*probability*) of a positive test result in a person with the disease or condition, or a measure of a test's ability to detect the disease correctly when the disease or condition is present. Also known as *true positive rate*.

Sensitivity analysis In *meta-analysis*, a method to check if a *pooled effect estimate* is *robust* to arbitrary methodological decisions made while compiling or analyzing the dataset used to conduct the meta-analysis.

Serial survey A survey that is administered with a certain periodicity, such as every five years. These surveys highlight change in patterns over time when comparing one period with another or several consecutive periods.

Serial time In the context of *survival analysis*, the amount of time between an individual entering a study and either the observation of an *event* of interest (failure) or *data censoring*.

Significance level See "*alpha*" (α).

Simple linear regression A linear regression model describing the relationship between two variables—one continuous *dependent variable* and one *independent variable*. See *linear regression*.

Simple logistic regression A *logistic regression* model describing the relationship between two variables—one categorical *dependent variable* and one *independent variable*. See *logistic regression*.

Simple randomization A method to generate a random sequence in which study participants are allocated to study arms randomly by using simple methods such as tossing a coin, rolling a die, or referencing a random number table.

Stratified randomization A method to randomly allocate study participants to study arms in which a study sample is split up or stratified by one or a few known *prognostic factors*. Study participants are then randomized within these strata. This method preemptively fixes the distribution of these important *prognostic factors* and between study arms and reduces the *probability* that by chance the groups will be imbalanced with regard to known *prognostic factors*.

Simple random sampling Methods to draw a sample using methods such as tossing a coin, rolling a die, or referencing a random number table.

Snowball sampling Sampling method that benefits from enrolled individuals inviting their peers satisfying the eligibility criteria for the study.

Specification See *restriction*.

Specificity The chance (probability) of a negative test result in a person without the disease or condition, or a measure of a test's ability to detect the absence of the disease or condition correctly when the disease or condition is absent. The percentage of all true negative test results among all people without the disease or condition (true negative + false positive). Also known as *true negative rate*.

Split-body randomized controlled trial (RCT) A RCT where an individual's body parts are randomized to study arms, such as a split-mouth trial.

Spread The quantification of how close together or far apart observed data are to a point estimate. Also known as dispersion or variability. Measures of spread include ranges, *quartiles*, *standard deviations*, and *variances*.

Spurious association Misleading association between two variables that appears to be related but is actually due to other factors (e.g., confounding) or random chance.

Standard deviation The average difference between each collected score and the mean that we would expect from a random sample of equal size drawn from the same population. It is measured in the original units of the data. A standard deviation of a sample is usually abbreviated as s, sd, std.dev or SD, and for a population as σ ("sigma"). Also known as variability. Standard deviation summarizes the variability of data, while standard error is a measure of precision and is meant to provide an estimate of a *population parameter* from a *sample statistic* in terms of the confidence *interval*.

Standard error (SE) The *standard deviation* of the *distribution* of means; a measure of how much the statistic varies from *sample* to sample; the standard error can be calculated as the standard deviation of the *sampling distribution*.

Standard error of the mean (SEM) A *standard error* calculated from sample *means*.

Standard error of a sample proportion A *standard error* calculated from sample proportions.

Standard error of the estimate Reflects the *variability* around the estimated regression line and the *accuracy* of the regression model.

Standard error of measurement Reflects the *variability* of the measurement error of a test and is often reported in standardized testing.

Standardize See *normalize*.

Standardized mean difference (SMD) or standardized difference in means A measure of association and summary statistics often used in *meta-analysis* when the included studies all assess the same *outcome* construct but measure it using different scales.

Standard normal distribution A normal distribution where the *frequency* distribution of scores surrounds a mean of "0" and a standard deviation of "1."; often referred to as a z distribution.

Statistical interaction See *effect modification*.

Statistical model Series of methods to collect, organize, analyze, interpret, and present data based on mathematical expressions.

Statistical significance Obtaining a *p-value* that is below the prespecified *level of significance* ("alpha"—α).

Statistics Statistics is a homonym with several meanings. 1) a number that is computed from data in a *sample* and can change from sample to sample. Also referred to as sample statistics. Sample statistics are denoted with Latin letters and mathematical symbols, e.g. x (x-bar) = sample mean, s or SD = standard deviation; 2) a discipline; 3) methods used to collect, synthesize, or interpret *quantitative data*; 4) metrics generated by statistical methods.

Stratification A strategy to deal with *confounding* in the analysis phase of a study where investigators separate the study participants into small subgroups or strata according to the potential *confounding variable*.

Stratified sampling A sampling method where a specific variable of interest, such as gender, is specific to nonoverlapping groups or strata. In other words, investigators divide the entire *population* of interest into two groups, such as males and females, and draw a *random sample* within each group or stratum.

Study arm Group of individuals in a *clinical trial* receiving an *intervention* of interest or a comparator.

Study population Individuals who are eligible for inclusion into a particular study. This is the population from which a *sample* is drawn for inclusion into the study.

Study results See *results*.

Systematic error See *bias*.

Systematic sampling A *sampling* method where individuals are selected using a specific unit of sampling. For example, out of 1,000 eligible individuals numbered from 1 to 1,000, researchers can determine to systematically select one participant for every 20 individuals.

Subgroup analysis In *meta-analysis*, a method to statistically assess if there are between-study (aggregated-level data) differences in effect estimates according to a particular attribute of interest. In *randomized controlled trials*, a method to statistically assess if within-study (individual-level data) differences in effect estimates exist according to an attribute of interest.

Subgroup effect See *effect modification*.

Summary effect estimate See *pooled effect estimate*.

Summary statistics See *descriptive statistics*.

Surrogate outcomes Outcomes that are precursors, predictors, or proxies of clinical- or *patient-important outcomes*.

Survival analysis A method to analyze outcome data that accounts for the time elapsed before an event of interest occurred. Also known as *time-to-event analysis*.

Survival curve A graphical representation of the progress of a *study population* over time. Starting from 100% survival rate (no participants experiencing the event of interest), the curve reflects the *event rate* over time until all individuals have experienced the event of interest or *censoring* data has occurred.

Survival time Event-free time period ending when the *event* of interest is observed (often an undesirable event).

Survival rate Proportion of participants in a study not experiencing the *event* of interest (often an undesirable event) over everyone exposed to the treatment or *prognostic factor*, at a given time. It is the opposite of the *hazard rate*.

Systematic error Errors that will affect all values, due to, for example, inaccurate measurement tools, using wrong units, or other methodological flaws. Also known as *bias*.

Systematic review A type of secondary research in which a focused research question drives the search, selection, appraisal, and synthesis of the results from primary studies from the research literature. Systematic reviews can be accompanied by a *meta-analysis*.

t-distribution A continuous bell-shaped like distribution. It is used when the population standard deviation is unknown or when the sample size is small.

t-statistic The test statistic derived from sample data after performing a t-test. The t-statistic follows a *t-distribution* under the *null hypothesis*.

Target population The entire group of individuals that a researcher wants to draw conclusions or make inferences about.

Tau squared A value quantifying the *between-study variance* or *heterogeneity* in the context of a meta-analysis. Typically abbreviated as the square of the Greek letter "τ" (tau)—τ^2.

Temporality bias See *antecedent consequence bias*.

Test accuracy Proportion of the sum of true positive test results and true negative results to the sum of all test results (sum of true positive, true negative, false positive and false negative results) when the test is used in a specified *population*.

Test-retest reliability A measure of how consistent the results of a measurement or a test is when repeated at different times. It is derived by repeating the measurement or test more than once over a period of time assuming that the measured attribute has not changed.

Test hypothesis See *alternative hypothesis*.

Test statistic A standardized value derived from sample data after performing a *hypothesis test*. It represents the distance between the data observed and the model prediction, such as the *null hypothesis*.

Time-to-event analysis See *survival analysis*.

Treatment effect A value used to quantify the impact of an intervention. This is different from an *effect size*, which quantifies the strength of a relationship between two *variables* or the difference between the values of two variables or groups in a standardized manner.

True negative rate (TNR) See *specificity*.

True positive rate (TPR) See *sensitivity*.

Type I error Rejecting a *null hypothesis* when the null hypothesis should not be rejected (a false positive determination). In other words, rejecting the null hypothesis when there is no difference (concluding that there is a difference when none exists).

Type II error Not rejecting the null hypothesis when it should be rejected (a false negative determination). In other words, not rejecting the null hypothesis when there is a difference (concluding there is no difference when a difference does exist).

Unbiased estimate *Effect estimate* that doesn't deviate from the true *population parameter.*

Validity Is the extent to which a questionnaire, instrument or tool (e.g., *a patient-reported outcome measure*) actually measures the underlying *construct* that is intended to measure.

Variable Any characteristics, number, or quantity of an individual that can be codified, measured or counted, and can take more than one value; any characteristic of an entity that can be measured (e.g. weight) or categorized (e.g. gender). When the variable of interest addresses the effects or consequences of an *intervention* or *exposure*, the variable is called *outcome.* See *binary or dichotomous variable, categorical or qualitative variable, continuous variable, discrete variable,* and *numeric or quantitative variable.*

Variability See *spread.*

Variance The *mean* squared deviation from the mean effect. The population variance is typically abbreviated as σ^2 ("sigma squared"), and the sample variance is typically abbreviated as s^2. The square of the original unit is the unit of the variance.

Weighted Obtaining an overall result by assigning different contributions (importance) to data points in a dataset.

Wilcoxon test In the context of survival analysis, a statistical test to compare two or more survival curves. This test emphasizes distances between the curves at the beginning of the curve (early on in the study).

Within-study variance The *variance* within each study in a *meta-analysis*; calculated by raising the *standard error* to the second power in the denominator.

Worst-case scenario analysis Conservative approach to assess the impact of missing data on study results, especially when evaluating an undesirable outcome. Individuals lost to follow-up in the intervention arm are analyzed as if they experienced the event of interest in the analysis and individuals lost to follow-up in the control arm are analyzed as if they did not experience the event of interest.

z-score A standard score which allows for calculations of the *probability* of a score within a normal distribution and enables comparisons of two scores from different normal distributions.

Index

Page locators in *italics* indicate figures and/or tables. Index terms in **bold** indicate there is also a glossary entry for this term. This index uses letter-by-letter alphabetization.

Statistics for Dental Clinicians, First Edition. Michael Glick, Alonso Carrasco-Labra, and Olivia Urquhart.
© 2024 John Wiley & Sons, Inc. Published 2024 by John Wiley & Sons, Inc.